SO-BRP-507

PRAISE FOR *THE BEST PRACTICE*

"*The Best Practice* is a timely and important contribution to the nation's ongoing struggle to make the best in modern health care available and affordable for all Americans. Charles Kenney introduces us to the pioneers at the forefront of this movement, highlighting the remarkable progress they are making, and illuminating the challenges that remain as they strive to improve the quality of health care in communities across the country."
—Senator Edward Kennedy

"*The Best Practice* argues persuasively that, in fact, getting sick in the United States doesn't beat getting sick in Sweden—or in Denmark, England, Germany, Canada, or just about anywhere else in the developed world, for that matter." —*Physicians Practice*

"*The Best Practice* is an amazingly readable book. My amazement is not a reflection on Kenney's writing, but rather that he managed to make health care quality interesting for nearly 300 pages."
—*TheHealthCareBlog.com*

"The quality movement in healthcare did not just happen on its own. It is the result of the insights, intelligence, idealism, creativity, and resilience of a handful of heroes. *The Best Practice* is their story, and Charles Kenney tells it in fast-paced, absorbing prose."
—Thomas H. Lee, M.D., network president
of Partners Healthcare System, and professor
of medicine at Harvard Medical School

"[Kenney's] telling of the health care quality movement has all the elements of a great story—human interest, compassion, inspiration, drama, and valuable insights into one of the most significant causes of our age."

—Helen Bevan, director of service transformation, NHS Institute for Innovation and Improvement

The Best Practice illuminate[s] how we can all work towards the goal of high-quality health care for all Americans. For those of us committed to achieving this goal in our lifetimes, this book shows us how much we need the visionaries profiled in these pages."

—Risa Lavizzo-Mourey, M.D., M.B.A., president and CEO, Robert Wood Johnson Foundation

The Best Practice is a must-read for anyone who cares about the state of American medicine. . . . [It] provides much-needed understanding of the complexity of ensuring the delivery of reliable, consistent, and high-quality medical care [and] shows how even small design flaws within the system can have serious ramifications for patient safety and care."

—Marshall N. Carter, former CEO, State Street Bank and Trust

THE BEST PRACTICE

THE BEST PRACTICE

How the New Quality Movement
Is Transforming Medicine

CHARLES KENNEY

PUBLICAFFAIRS
NEW YORK

Copyright © 2008 by Charles Kenney

Hardcover edition first published in 2008 in the United States by PublicAffairs™,
A Member of the Perseus Books Group.
Paperback edition first published in 2010 in the United States by PublicAffairs

All rights reserved.
Printed in the United States of America.

No part of this book may be reproduced in any manner whatsoever without written
permission except in the case of brief quotations embodied in critical articles and
reviews. For information, address PublicAffairs, 250 West 57th Street, Suite 1321,
New York, NY 10107.

PublicAffairs books are available at special discounts for bulk purchases in the U.S. by
corporations, institutions, and other organizations. For more information, please contact
the Special Markets Department at the Perseus Books Group, 2300 Chestnut Street,
Suite 200, Philadelphia, PA 19103, call (800) 810-4145, extension 5000, or e-mail
special.markets@perseusbooks.com.

Designed by Linda Harper
Text set in Fairfield LH Light

A CIP catalog record for this book is available from the Library of Congress

HC ISBN: 978-1-58648-619-8
PB ISBN: 978-1-58648-797-3

10 9 8 7 6 5 4 3 2

Robert Mandel, MD, MBA,
deserves particular recognition for his contribution to this book.
Robert combines clinical knowledge and experience along with
acumen on the business side of health care. Throughout the process
he has served as a teacher, sounding board, and guide.
He read several drafts of the manuscript and offered
important suggestions and guidance. I am very grateful to him.

This book is for the caregivers, patients and families
who are showing the way to improved quality.

Contents

CONTENTS

Foreword

Call to Action

This book is about solving one of the most difficult, complicated, and critical problems facing our country today. For years, the collapse of our health care system has been predicted so persistently and pervasively that many people have become immune to the warning. Others have decided that we should just abandon the current system altogether. As you see in these pages, however, there is a growing cadre of people—leaders in health care, business and academia—who are engaged in transforming the system so that it provides safe, timely, effective, and affordable patient-centered care for everyone.

Theirs is a heroic effort. Not only are they immediately saving lives and improving the health of patients, they are also building an entirely new framework for the delivery of health care. They are working toward the day when medical miracles are not just available to the few but are accessible to all, and when every doctor's office is a center of clinical excellence. This is achievable, imperative, and, I believe, inevitable.

Certainly, the transformation of our health care system is long overdue. It has been seven years since the Institute of Medicine concluded that we experience as many as 98,000 preventable patient deaths in the U.S. health care system every year. That is more than 250 preventable deaths a day, year in and year out. Would any other system, industry, or enterprise in the United States accept, or be allowed, such errors? As a community, how long should we endure this loss and suffering? We must not lose sight of the real people behind these numbers.

This is not simply a clinical problem or the result of incompetent physicians. As Dr. Donald Berwick, President and Chief Executive Officer of the Institute for Healthcare Improvement, has said: "The vast majority of medical mistakes are committed not by bad apples, but by good doctors trying to do the right thing, working under conditions that do not account for the fact that they are human." It is a fragmented and poorly designed system we have inherited and unconsciously nurtured that perpetuates medical errors and leads to the misuse, overuse, and underuse of health care.

The facts speak for themselves. For example, we are uncertain about the clinical benefit of almost half the care we provide in our country. Most of the care we receive is not based on randomized clinical trials. In fact, only about 20 percent has been scientifically tested. It has been estimated that a quarter of all new drug prescriptions contain errors. Even more disturbing is that the United States ranks only twenty-third among industrialized nations in infant mortality rates, yet we spend about 16 percent of our Gross Domestic Product (GDP) on health care.

In my state, Massachusetts, the Commonwealth Fund determined that just over 50 percent of diabetics receive recommended care, and Massachusetts ranked thirty-fifth in the nation on avoidable hospital use and costs. Our own Department of Public Health found that hospital-acquired infections may cost the Massachusetts health care system as much as $473 million a year, not to mention the dire health risk these infections pose for the affected patients.

All of us who work in the health care system are accountable for these results. Even health care payers, such as the health insurance plan I lead in Massachusetts, must take responsibility and a leading position in the transformation of our health care system. We must change what is a perverse payment system into one that supports the efforts of people like those described in these pages. As long as physicians and hospitals can only improve their bottom lines by conducting more visits, more tests, and more surgeries rather than by providing better health outcomes for patients, we will continue to pay more and more for unacceptable care. We must insist that health care insurance premiums pay for the best possible care, not just volume. I believe that health care consultant and author Michael Millenson put it best when he answered the question: If more care isn't better, what is? Millenson said, "Better care is better." And, I believe, a system that demands better health outcomes will not only save lives, but will also go far to rein in the unsustainable trend in health care costs. The health care quality movement thought leaders and pioneers cited in this book are showing us the way to a transformed health care system. Here, I offer my thoughts on some essential principles for achieving the health care system we want.

We should demand:

- A system with a goal of "zero preventable harm" for each and every patient
- All patients receive appropriate and evidence-based care, whether preventive or for acute or chronic conditions
- A system that eliminates racial and cultural disparities in access to, and the delivery of, health care
- Those who deliver care are rewarded on the basis of objective performance measures related to the quality of clinical outcomes

- Patients receive what they need to make informed choices
- Health system leaders, especially trustees and board members of hospitals and health care companies, become strong and consistent advocates of quality on behalf of those they serve
- New technologies and treatments are evaluated and compared to existing alternatives prior to their adoption
- The public and health care providers are fully informed about opportunities for improving care
- Savings from a safer, more evidence-based and cost-effective health care system are reinvested in a way that slows the spiraling cost of health care and improves the health of the community.

Almost every day, we hear about efforts, old and new, to conquer disease, save lives, and improve personal health and quality of life. We have the science. We have the medical expertise. We have the technology and managerial competency. We have dedicated and impassioned people who stand ready to deliver on the promise of twenty-first-century medicine. Now, we must provide the will and motivation to transform our health care system into one that realizes our highest aspirations for health care.

Cleve L. Killingsworth
CHAIRMAN AND CHIEF EXECUTIVE OFFICER
BLUE CROSS BLUE SHIELD OF MASSACHUSETTS

THE BEST PRACTICE

Introduction: Betsy Lehman

*"If this can happen at
a place like Dana-Farber . . . "*

On a sunny autumn day in October 1994, Betsy Lehman hurried through the bustling newsroom of the *Boston Globe*. She was petite, with large, sparkling eyes, and although she was thirty-nine she could easily have passed for a graduate student. Betsy resembled a pretty version of Annie from the Broadway show—curly-haired, wholesome, all-American. A Phi Beta Kappa graduate of Brown University, she had proved her mettle as a dependable general assignment reporter before earning a promotion to chief medical columnist—one of the most prestigious beats at the paper. She was known for her infectious energy, compassion, and insightful intellect. Betsy had worked the medical beat for eight of her twelve years at the *Globe,* writing about the most elusive medical concepts with style and clarity, and earning widespread respect throughout the city's exacting medical community.

As she approached the message center near the heart of the *Globe* newsroom, Rose Devine, one of the telephone operators, called out to her—"Betsy, your hair looks great!" "Thanks, Rose," Betsy replied with a rueful smile. "It's a wig." She shrugged and added: "Chemo."

For a few minutes, Betsy stood by the message center chatting with several colleagues who had gathered around her. They all knew she'd been waging a battle against breast cancer for more than a year, ever since she had been diagnosed in September 1993. Subsequently, she had undergone a standard treatment—surgery followed by about six months of chemotherapy. Although this regimen had proved quite effective for many patients, it had not worked for Betsy. The cancer spread to her lungs, and she required a considerably more aggressive and much riskier form of treatment. Researchers in Boston and elsewhere feverishly generated promising new treatments, some of which were in clinical trials. A few of the trials would work, many (perhaps most) would not, and it was far from clear during the early stages which was which. Betsy's doctors would guide her, but the decision on which treatment to choose would ultimately rest with her.

As daunting as the situation was, it would have been difficult to imagine a person better positioned to deal with it than Betsy. She seemed to know just about everybody in Boston's sprawling medical community, affording her easy access to some of the finest medical minds in the world. This was her business, after all; this was what she did—examining, studying, questioning, probing, sifting through the latest medical protocols and treatments. Her skill at understanding medical complexities and translating them into straightforward language had helped countless readers navigate the daunting medical landscape. She would now have to use that skill to try to save her own life.

Yet another advantage was Betsy's husband's affiliation with Dana-Farber Cancer Institute, where he worked as a cancer researcher. Dana-Farber is a Harvard teaching hospital with a well-earned reputation as one of the finest cancer centers in the world. Boston is home to other world-class hospitals, of course—Massachusetts

General, Brigham and Women's, Beth Israel-Deaconess, Children's, New England Medical Center, Boston Medical Center, and more. And although all offer top-notch cancer services, Dana-Farber specializes in cancer—that is their only business—the sole source of their research and clinical service. The institute's founder, Dr. Sidney Farber, was a key figure in the invention of chemotherapy, and Baruj Benacerraf, the former president, was awarded a Nobel Prize in Medicine in 1980.

Betsy entered Dana-Farber on November 14, 1994, for chemotherapy and a bone marrow transplant, an aggressive new approach that seemed to offer hope. There was no doubt that the treatment would be punishing, perhaps brutal; but as the mother of two little girls, Emily Claire, aged seven, and Laura Margaret, aged three, what choice did she have? Before being admitted, Betsy had written an e-mail to a friend who also had cancer: "I personally see being at my children's birthdays as a triumph. May we both see our kids' cakes crowded with many, many candles." And later: "I guess I'm resigned to the idea of going through hell for the hope of a chance."

No sooner had the chemotherapy commenced, however, when Betsy's body ballooned, swelling in grotesque fashion even as she was overwhelmed by wracking bouts of vomiting. "She was dealing with horrendous symptoms," her husband would later tell the *Boston Globe*. "The whole lining of her gut from one end to the other was shedding. She was vomiting sheets of tissue. . . . But the doctors said this was all normal with bone marrow transplants." It was so bad at one point that Betsy asked a nurse: "Am I going to die from vomiting?"

But in the eyes of the staff at Dana-Farber, Betsy's reaction to the drugs was not altogether out of the ordinary. They dealt with extreme reactions to treatments every day. And in the coming weeks, it appeared the treatment was working—the transplanted cells were doing what they were supposed to do, and after three weeks of treatment Betsy was scheduled to go home on Saturday,

December 3. That morning, however, she was profoundly unsettled. A nurse characterized her as "weepy, anxious this A.M. regarding discharge home before she is ready." She left a phone message for a friend, saying in part: "I'm feeling very frightened, very upset. I don't know what's wrong, but something's wrong."

Soon after leaving the phone message, Betsy collapsed in her room and could not be resuscitated. Shortly after noon, Betsy Amanda Lehman died. She was thirty-nine.

Betsy's obituary noted that she died "while undergoing treatment for breast cancer," and that, of course, was true, but it did not tell the real story, nor even hint at the unthinkable dimensions of the tragedy. More than two months passed before the truth emerged, finding its way into daylight by happenstance. On February 13, 1995, an assistant data manager was reviewing piles of numbers on the hospital's many clinical trials when she unearthed a horrific error: Dana-Farber had mistakenly given Betsy a massive drug overdose. A doctor wrote an order indicating 6,520 milligrams of Cytoxan—a number he intended as a total dose over four days. Nurses and pharmacists, however, read the number as the dose to be administered on *each* of the four days. Thus, while Betsy was supposed to receive 1,630 milligrams of the exceptionally powerful drug each day for four days, she actually received four times that— 6,520 milligrams per day for four days. The dosage overwhelmed her strong heart, killing her.

It turned out that Betsy was not the only victim of a chemotherapy overdose at Dana-Farber at the time. Maureen Bateman, a fifty-two-year-old patient, was administered a comparable overdose weeks before Betsy's treatment. Mrs. Bateman's heart was irreversibly damaged, yet she survived for three more years until her death at the age of fifty-five.

In the shock that followed Betsy's death the questions were obvious: How could such a mistake happen at one of the premier cancer centers in the world? How could such an egregious error have been made in the first place and, once made, how was it possible that other experienced professionals—doctors, nurses, and pharmacists—had failed to catch it? The anger of Betsy's friends and colleagues at the *Globe* was reflected in the newspaper's editorial: "Betsy's heart stopped after a massive overdose of an anticancer drug, inexplicably quadrupled beyond the normally prescribed amounts. It was an error so glaring that any first-year medical student should have spotted it, and yet the country's top specialists, pharmacists and nurses let it slip by."

This tragic mistake would have been stunning in any hospital anywhere in the country, but the fact that it had occurred in Boston, of all places, was doubly disturbing. For Boston was a city where brilliant clinicians and researchers were drawn to great hospitals, medical schools, and universities; a city that defined itself in large measure based on its medical achievements and reputation. Dr. O. Michael Colvin, then at Johns Hopkins University School of Medicine, now director emeritus, Duke University Comprehensive Cancer Center, got to the heart of the matter. "It frightens me," he said. "If this can happen at a place like Dana-Farber, a nationally respected institute, what is happening in other places?"

Betsy's death made national news. Soon after the true cause of death was revealed, *Time* magazine published "The Disturbing Case of the Cure That Killed the Patient." The article observed that Betsy's case was one among a number of others, including instances in which a patient in Florida had the wrong leg amputated and a woman in Michigan had the wrong breast removed. "Are these isolated, if horrifying, events? Or could they be harbingers of a deadly trend?" the *Time* article asked. *Time* noted that "even the most routine procedures can go awry." In late March 1995, just a week before the *Time* article was published, a four-year-old girl had died after undergoing a tonsillectomy. The magazine observed:

Like 100,000 other Americans each year, Desiree Wade was sent home a few hours after the surgery. . . . She developed a fever and became increasingly sick. Her coughs apparently tore open the surgical wounds in her throat, and she bled to death. If a tonsillectomy can go bad, imagine all the things that can happen with a bone-marrow transplant, a coronary-bypass operation, or an experiment in gene therapy. As medicine has become more complex and the pace of technological change has accelerated, the opportunities for error have multiplied.

Investigations were launched as Dana-Farber administrators disciplined several doctors and pharmacists. The Joint Commission on Accreditation of Healthcare Organizations, America's leading hospital regulatory body, placed Dana-Farber on probation, an incredible humiliation for such a distinguished institution. Within a year came a house-cleaning and thorough management shake-up.

Most clinicians saw Betsy's death as a straightforward case of human error: A fatal mistake had been made and no one had picked up on it. Many doctors and nurses privately whispered: "There but for the grace of God go I." *And they meant it.* They knew that sort of mistake could have been made by *anyone*—by the most brilliant among them. Many clinicians wondered whether the chemotherapy instructions were as clear as they could have been. The order was for "cyclophosphamide dose 4 grams/square meter (of body surface area) over 4 days." Was that four grams total in four days? Or four grams each day for four days? The fellow administering the medicine incorrectly read it as the latter. Finger pointing and recriminations soon followed—administrators were fired, doctors, nurses, and pharmacists disciplined. The implication was that by ridding the system of people who had made mistakes, excellence would be restored.

But would an administrative shuffle really solve the problem? And more to the point, what, exactly, *was* the problem? Was it one incompetent doctor who had erred on the dosage? But how could one doctor making a single mistake so completely penetrate safeguards—enough to kill a patient? Many others—doctors, nurses, and pharmacists—participated in the treatment. Were *all* of these doctors, nurses, and pharmacists incompetent? Were *all* poorly trained? *All* insufficiently dedicated? At the time, Dana-Farber included some of the most dedicated men and women anywhere in the field of medicine—well-educated and trained, hard-working, and passionately devoted to their patients.

Still, there had been a fatal error.

Since the time of Hippocrates more than 2,500 years ago, the men and women who devote their lives to medicine have aspired to the highest possible standards of quality. Each and every day in the United States and throughout the world there are countless examples of outstanding, even heroic, efforts to care for patients. There have been hundreds, thousands, of such examples through the years at Dana-Farber alone.

In spite of all that, however, the scientific evidence now points to the inescapable conclusion that American health care is deeply flawed. Research reveals that, in spite of the competence and dedication of clinicians, American health care is plagued by a quality deficiency. Two of the most intellectually distinguished organizations in the United States affirm this conclusion. The RAND Corporation is one of the premier research organizations in the world, renowned for its work in a variety of complex fields. RAND found that Americans—regardless of race, ethnicity or socioeconomic status—receive the right care (the consensus scientific care for their condition) only about half the time. RAND concluded that "everyone is at risk of receiving poor care, no matter what their condition, where they live, from whom they seek care, or what their gender, race, or financial status is."

It is critical to understand that quality is not defined as having access to the prominent orthopedic surgeon, nor admission to a "name" hospital. Nor is quality merely the absence of error. Quality care is, by definition, error free, but the definition of quality care is far broader. The Institute of Medicine of the National Academies defines quality as care that is safe, effective, efficient, equitable, patient-centered, and timely. Quality care is evidence-based care; care that is based on scientific study identifying the best treatment possible. Quality care occurs when patients "get the care that the medical evidence has shown will benefit them based on their diagnosis and condition and that they do not receive care where the potential for harm outweighs the benefit."

Two of the nation's leading academic experts on health care, professors Michael E. Porter and Elizabeth Olmstead Teisberg, have written in their book *Redefining Health Care* that "in the past two decades, health care has gone from being a source of national pride to one of America's preeminent concerns."

Landmark studies from the Institute of Medicine (IOM) conclude that millions of patients who would benefit from widely recognized and available treatments do not get those treatments; that millions more receive medications or treatments known to have no effective impact; and that millions of preventable errors are committed each year resulting in as many as 98,000 hospital patient deaths. One of the most significant quality assessments during the last twenty-five years was done by the Institute of Medicine— *Crossing the Quality Chasm: A New Health System for the 21st Century.* Published in 2001, the report's findings remain as cogent today as ever:

Health care today harms too frequently and routinely fails to deliver its potential benefits. Americans should be able to count on receiving care that meets their needs and is based on the best scientific knowledge. Yet there is strong evidence that this frequently is not the case. Crucial reports from disciplined review bodies document the scale and gravity of the problem. Quality problems are everywhere. . . . *Between the health care we have and the health care we could have lies not just a gap, but a chasm* (emphasis added).

Dr. Steven A. Schroeder, Distinguished Professor of Health and Health Care at the University of California–San Francisco, wrote in the *New England Journal of Medicine* that "the United States spends more on health care than any other nation in the world, yet it ranks poorly on nearly every measure of health status . . . too many Americans do not receive [needed care], receive it too late, or receive poor-quality care." Dr. Schroeder notes that "among the 30 developed nations that make up the Organization for Economic Cooperation and Development (OECD), the United States ranks near the bottom on most standard measures of health status." In another measure comparing countries throughout the world the U.S. ranks forty-second in infant mortality and forty-sixth in life expectancy.

Even a casual glance at the findings from RAND, IOM, and other credible sources makes clear that in America today too many patients are harmed; too many killed; too many fail to get the right care. And the scandal in American medicine today is that too little is being done about it. RAND findings indicate the scope of the quality gap in the United States. For example, diabetic patients receive slightly less than half the care they need, and hypertension patients get less than 65 percent of care recommended for their illness. Preventive care is an essential element of quality care, yet throughout the United States we fall far well short of prescribed and desirable preventive care. In a study of 300 managed care plans, RAND found that more than one-third of the children did *not* receive recommended immunizations by age two—truly fundamental elements of quality care.

Donald M. Berwick, a Harvard-trained physician and CEO of the Institute for Healthcare Improvement, says flatly: "The myth that America has the best health care in the world is just that—a myth."

Yet this sweeping indictment speaks not to uncaring, poorly trained doctors and nurses. In the United States, we are blessed with some of the most committed clinicians in the world. Rather, these findings illustrate the woefully inconsistent nature of the health care delivery *system,* a system that often handcuffs clinicians. "Health care has safety and quality problems because it relies on outmoded systems of work," found the IOM. "Poor designs set the workforce up to fail, —regardless of how hard they try. If we want safer, higher-quality care, we will need to have redesigned systems of care." RAND agreed: "To substantially improve the quality of health care available to all patients, we need to focus on large-scale, *systemwide* changes."

A number of scientists have conducted quantitative comparisons between performance in health care and other high-risk industries. Roger Resar, MD, a senior fellow at the Institute for Healthcare Improvement, has compared health care to both the airline and nuclear power industries, and he estimates that, in health care delivery, defects (failing to administer the correct dosage of medication, for example) occur 10 to 20 percent of the time. With airlines and nuclear power plants, the defect rate is 1 in 10,000.

A significant part of the quality problem can be traced to the surprising and entirely counterintuitive fact that, in health care, *performance is rarely measured.* Although nearly everything else of significance in the world of the twenty-first century is measured, health care is the surprising exception. Economic measurements abound with companies graded in hundreds of ways, including a daily share price calculation. Major industrial corporations measure every aspect of their design, production, distribution, and sales processes. A fantasy baseball league participant making decisions on which players to select has more data—by an order of magnitude—

than a patient choosing a brain or heart surgeon. Yet hospitals don't even measure who the best cancer surgeons are.

Clinicians at Cincinnati Children's Hospital, an outstanding institution in so many respects, believed they were among the finest cystic fibrosis centers in the country; but when the Cystic Fibrosis Foundation measured performance, the folks in Cincinnati were dumbstruck to learn they ranked near the bottom. Many hospitals and physician groups that believe they are delivering quality care are failing to do so. They don't know the work is poor because they are not measured. It is, at the very least, ironic that an industry populated by very bright men and women who have been measured throughout their academic careers—and achieved lofty results along the way—escape most measurement upon entering practice.

Professors Porter and Teisberg write that *"mandatory measurement and reporting of results is perhaps the single most important step in reforming the health care system"* (emphasis in original).

Why is measurement so critical? Because clinicians don't know what needs improvement until they measure. If patients wanted to seed a grassroots revolution in health care they would demand, above all else, measurement—for measurement would tell them who to see for a particular operation or treatment and who to avoid. Measurement would tell every clinician and hospital where they rank and what they need to do to get better.

George Halvorson, chairman and CEO of Kaiser Permanente, one of the largest integrated health care organizations in the country, believes measurement can transform medicine. "Health care measures almost nothing when judged by the normal standards of performance tracking that exist for any category of systematic quality improvement processes used by other major industries," Halvorson observes. Halvorson says patients need to know whether "one oncology group had a 90 percent five-year survival rate for Stage 1A breast cancer, and another group down the street had [a 40 percent survival rate]."

Although the lack of measurement is a central cause of the quality chasm, so, too, is the sparse use in American health care of information technology—the kind of IT that is standard in every other major industry in the world. Tens of millions of paper files in medical offices are a vivid indicator of how far behind other industries health care is in terms of information technology. Advanced information technology incorporates the very latest scientific information to aid doctors in diagnosing and treating disease. Programs enable physicians to load symptoms into the computer and receive an array of data that provide invaluable assistance to the doctor in diagnosing and treating. Yet the great majority of doctors in the United States today do *not* have such technology at their disposal.

Technology is also essential to enabling doctors to keep up with the avalanche of new scientific information each year. As the *Chasm* report notes: "No doctor—no matter how brilliant, dedicated and skilled—could possibly keep abreast of all the latest medical advances. . . . Weed has pointed out that to ask an individual practitioner to rely on his or her memory to store and retrieve all the facts relevant to patient care is like asking a travel agent to memorize airline schedules."

Betsy Lehman's daughter Emily Clare was seven when her mother died. She's twenty-one now, a student in college. Laura Margaret was three. She is a seventeen-year-old high school student. Betsy's husband, Bob Distel, remains on the job at Dana-Farber, devoted to his work seeking to conquer cancer.

The Institute of Medicine reports that every year anywhere from 44,000 to 98,000 Americans die from preventable medical errors. Since Betsy Lehman died, that translates into approximately 700,000 and 1,400,000 *preventable* deaths from medical errors in American hospitals. Consider the impact of these deaths—on children such as Emily Clare and Laura Margaret; on parents and siblings, spouses and friends. If one death devastates a family—a circle of family and friends—then what is the impact of a million such deaths? Beyond the deaths, *tens of millions* of Americans have been harmed by medical errors since Betsy died, and tens of millions more have not received the quality care they needed to maximize their health and well-being.

But change is coming to doctors' offices and hospitals throughout the country—change based on a recognition of the reality rather than the myth of American health care. And the change is rooted in a rock-solid commitment to safer, higher-quality care. Incremental change will not cut it, says William R. Brody, MD, PhD, president of Johns Hopkins University. "This," says Brody, "is a revolution."

And the revolution has grown into a powerful social movement in the United States and beyond. From the fringes it has barged into the mainstream of health care where it is, to some, deeply threatening; to others, it is something of a savior. It is a movement stirring fierce debate, and yet opposition at this point can only stall its progress rather than stop it altogether. The power of the movement—with an army of tens of thousands of clinicians, patients, policymakers, and academics—has gained enough sustained power to force its way into common practice. Although that will not happen overnight, it is in fact happening with warp speed in many places around the country and the world.

This book is, in part, about what's wrong with our health care system, but it is focused to a far greater degree on the burgeoning influence of the new quality movement. At its core, this book is about how the movement is transforming the way we deliver and manage care. This is the story of visionaries, mavericks, and revolutionaries with impeccable pedigrees and experience in some of the most prestigious hospitals in the world; the story of a small group of physicians and other scientists who see things others do not yet see; who believe what others have never imagined. At its core, this is the story of a small band of crusaders who have set out to change the medical world.

1

Early History of the
New Quality Movement

———∽∽∽∽———

"We gold-plated the bolt."

Dr. Donald M. Berwick never saw it coming. He had been through medical school, internship, and residency, and he had worked at the Harvard School of Public Health; now he was with the Harvard Community Health Plan (HCHP)—and never before had a colleague thrown anything at him.

It was 1982 and Berwick was a thirty-six-year-old doctor on a mission. As the director of quality assurance for the Harvard Community Health Plan in Boston, he was responsible for analyzing a variety of statistics designed to measure the plan's quality of care. The Harvard Plan, an HMO founded by the Harvard Medical School, had managed to get itself into financial difficulty and Berwick's job was to make sure that quality did not suffer even as significant budget cutbacks were imposed on operations. It was a tense time. Doctors didn't like the budget cuts, and they liked Berwick's monitoring even less. Berwick recalls the scope of the project—and the difficulties he encountered: "We measured infant mortality, infection rates, waiting times, failures to follow-up tests, endless numbers of measurements and endless conflict because the process itself was not welcome in the organization by the work force. After all, they are working as hard as they can and I'm showing up with reports saying that people are waiting too long, or that infections are up, or whatever."

Berwick and his team conducted detailed interviews with patients and scoured medical records. They noted patients who had had abnormal Pap smears, for example, and then determined what percent of those patients had undergone follow-up exams, something that should have been happening in 100 percent of the cases—true quality of care—and yet the reality was below that.

On the basis of this research, Berwick would rate each HCHP doctor on a variety of measures—the most detailed report card the doctors had likely received since medical school. "My aim was to begin to understand patterns of patient satisfaction at the individual doctor level from a random sample of every single doctor's patients," says Berwick.

Over time, Berwick and his team collected information from patients on scores of measures relating to about a hundred physicians, then reviewed and analyzed the data. Berwick assembled reports on each doctor, assigning a patient satisfaction score for everything from waiting times to follow-ups to the doctor's personal interaction with the patient. Finally, after months of work, Berwick stepped before a group of physicians, distributed the results, and started what he was sure would be an intense discussion of the material.

His first stop was the internal medicine group at the Kenmore Center, located in the shadow of Boston's Fenway Park. Two dozen or so doctors gathered in a conference room to hear Berwick's results.

Each doctor was given a sealed envelope containing the scores for every doctor in the room, identities disguised. No one knew who doctors A, B, or C were, but Berwick's staff had highlighted each physician's results so that the doctor would know his or her own scores and could measure them against the others.

This was a big moment for Berwick, the fruit of an enormous amount of labor. Don Berwick, a bespectacled dark-haired man of slim build, had a passion for his work. His hope was that the physicians would take the data to heart and use it to target areas for improvement. He saw it not only as a reality check but also as a motivational tool.

He stood at the front of the room exuding earnest intensity; yet, as he summarized the project and explained the scores, an unsettling air of tension pervaded the room. The doctors, Berwick knew, were well-trained, intelligent people who were deeply devoted to the practice of medicine. Like most physicians, they wanted to be left alone to do what they believed was best for their patients. But it was Berwick's job to question, quantify, measure, and analyze—and that is precisely what he had done.

When the material was distributed, the room fell silent save for the sound of envelopes being torn open and the rustling of paper as the doctors reviewed the data.

After about a minute, the physician farthest from Berwick rose from her seat and strode around the conference table to the front of the room. She took the report in her hands, crumpled it into a ball, and threw it at Don Berwick. And then, wordlessly, she was gone.

Don Berwick has come a long way since that day in Kenmore Square. In the ensuing twenty-five years, Berwick has led a health care crusade throughout the United States and far beyond. As one of the founders and now the CEO of the Institute for Healthcare Improvement in Cambridge, Massachusetts, Berwick has become synonymous with the new quality movement. Atul Gawande, MD, a Boston surgeon and *New Yorker* staff member, wrote that Berwick "is an unusual figure in medicine" in that "he is powerful not because of the position he holds. . . . He is powerful because of *how he thinks* [emphasis added]."

Berwick has been asked to advise health systems about quality from Australia to Israel and the Palestinian territories; from Malawi to Sweden, Dubai to the United Kingdom. Twice, the publication *Modern Healthcare* called him the third most influential individual in American health care. His honors speak volumes: quality and leadership awards from the American Hospital Association (AHA), the National Quality Forum, the Joint Commission, and, in 2005, a knighthood from Queen Elizabeth II. He is a fellow of the Royal College of Physicians of London and has been chosen to serve on a presidential commission on health care quality as well as on the two most important health care committees of the Institute of Medicine of the National Academies. He has produced hundreds of articles in journals ranging from *Pediatrics* to the *New England Journal of Medicine,* from *Quality Management in Health Care* to the *Journal of the American Medical Association* (*JAMA*). He serves on the faculties of Harvard's School of Public Health and Medical School and consults in pediatrics at Massachusetts General and Children's Hospitals.

In building the new quality movement, Berwick is joined by a growing number of impressively credentialed physicians, academics, administrators, and hospital trustees, all anchored by clinicians working on the front lines of medicine. Berwick has also gone beyond the boundaries of medicine in searching out techniques that will improve health care. He has committed the medically heretical act of enlisting some of the leading industrial quality-control engineers in the nation, namely, men and women whose expertise is creating industrial systems that minimize or even eliminate error in complex systems as they significantly improve quality. These are PhD engineers who work to perfect production systems for airlines and nuclear power stations as well as electronics and automobile manufacturers. From them Berwick learned that quality is created not by individuals alone but by individuals working within well-designed systems. He has used this lesson to transform the way we think about error in medicine, "complications," and what it means to receive true quality of care.

Berwick grew up in Moodus, Connecticut, a rural town in the south central portion of the state, where his father was one of two doctors in town, both with horse-and-buggy-type practices, which meant touring the area making house calls. "I was the doctor's son, and I don't ever remember not wanting to be a doctor," Berwick recalls. "I always knew I would be." Berwick's mother, who was active in a variety of town causes, including the synagogue, died when her son was just fifteen, but she left him with the strong impression that public service was a noble calling.

In a high school graduating class of just fifty-three students, Berwick was accepted to Harvard, which, he notes, was "quite an eye-opener for a small-town person." As a pre-med student he majored in a combination of psychology and sociology. (His first day of school at Harvard was undoubtedly his best. His biology lab partner that day, Ann Greenberg, later became his wife.) After graduating from Harvard in 1968 (summa cum laude, Phi Beta Kappa), Berwick had packed his bags for the trip to Yale when, at the last minute, he was told he'd been moved off the waiting list and admitted to Harvard Medical School. It was the Vietnam era, a time when protestors shut down universities and took to the streets. During his first year of medical school, Berwick was restless. "The science was great, but this was the era of politics and political awareness," he recalls. But he had trouble reconciling his active involvement in the antiwar movement with the absence of policy concerns in medicine. Then Berwick heard about a program at Harvard's John F. Kennedy School of Government that granted a joint degree in any one of various disciplines (medicine, business, or law, for example) as well as public policy. The faculty was distinguished, the classes small, the work intense—and Berwick loved it: "The content was analytic methods basically, operations research, statistics, political science, economics," he recalls. "The idea was to equip people from subject matter areas, like medicine, law, and engineering with knowledge of how public policy gets formulated, and should get formulated."

The public policy program was formative for Berwick, and would change the way he thought about medicine. He became familiar with the use of analytic techniques to study processes and systems, which, as he would later learn, quality in health was all about.

After medical school, Berwick began his training in internal medicine at Massachusetts General Hospital. Midway, he realized that his real passion lay in pediatrics, and he moved to Children's Hospital for pediatric training—his favorite medical school rotation— "taking care of kids with leukemia . . . using every single resource I had, everything—physical, mental—complete involvement. And it was great."

Berwick eventually found his way to the Harvard School of Public Health, where he worked until 1982, when he was hired by the Harvard Community Health Plan (HCHP). He was at HCHP on the unfortunate day when the well-meaning and carefully prepared report, its statistics and analysis having been so earnestly gathered, was balled up and hurled at him. He had had another dispiriting, though amusing, encounter around the same time. As he studied reams of statistics, he noticed that the radiology department had shown a sudden and rather dramatic improvement in waiting times. Berwick was both pleased by this and curious about how it had been achieved. He visited the department administrator and asked what process she had put in place to shorten waiting times so much.

Wellll . . . actually, she said, a bit sheepishly . . . the waiting times had not really improved—hadn't changed at all, as a matter of fact. Berwick was taken aback and told her about the new data indicating the shorter waits.

To Berwick's astonishment she looked at him and replied: "I lied. I just started making up data and sent it to you. You keep sending me these negative reports and I get in trouble and I'm trying as hard as I can to fix them. And I thought you'd be happier if I just told you everything was okay. I knew I'd be happier."

As difficult and unrewarding as his quality work was in those early days, Berwick was energized by the one day a week he spent seeing patients. An evaluation of Berwick's performance by superiors and colleagues yielded a comment from the chief of pediatrics that "never in conducting a review of a pediatrician have I received such uniformly laudatory comments."

Berwick was devoted to quality improvement, but it was a grind. After four years of difficult, frustrating work at the Harvard Plan, Berwick felt so discouraged that his impulse was to move on, but a conversation with Tom Pyle, the Harvard Plan CEO, changed his mind. Pyle's business experience was outside health care, and he told Berwick that certain businesses approached quality in a way that was quite different and perhaps more effective. Pyle urged Berwick to examine some of those approaches and decide whether any could be adapted to health care.

This was a critical moment, a test, of sorts, for Don Berwick. He was a product of a medical culture not unfamiliar with a tilt toward arrogance, one that suggested *we in medicine know best and people in other industries, well . . . let's just say they're not Harvard-trained doctors.* This thick crust of hubris on the medical profession, which often insulated doctors from better ideas elsewhere, might well have prevented other doctors from following Tom Pyle's advice. But Don Berwick has the keen ability to listen with an open mind and to recognize good ideas whatever their origin, attributes that enabled Berwick to shift gears and begin his search for quality outside of health care. It was a search that would fundamentally alter the direction not only of Berwick's life but of health care in the United States.

After some quick research, Berwick identified several organizations as having particularly strong reputations for quality, among them NASA, Bell Laboratories, Gillette, and Toyota stood out in particular. Berwick decided to start with NASA. (This was, of course, before the *Challenger* disaster.) It was 1985 when Berwick met with Haggai (Guy) Cohen, the director of reliability, quality, and safety, Office of Manned Space Flight. When Berwick explained who he was and what he was up to, Guy Cohen was immediately curious to know more about why a medical doctor was interested in the NASA quality systems. He offered to come up from Washington to talk about quality face-to-face.

Not long afterward, Cohen arrived at the Harvard Community Health Plan office at the Kenmore Center, unpacked more than 300 acetate transparencies, and proceeded to walk Berwick through the system of management NASA used to ensure quality. Guy Cohen was an unassuming, middle-aged engineer with a soft voice and affable manner. Yet there was a steeliness about him, a sense of rock-solid confidence when he spoke about management processes designed to yield quality outcomes at NASA.

The first statement he made to Berwick was straightforward: "I'm the head of quality, safety, and reliability at NASA. I report to the administrator of NASA, and the administrator reports to the president of the United States." Recalls Berwick: "He wasn't puffing, this wasn't a power move. He was saying, 'What I do is regarded in my system as extremely important.'" Berwick thought, "Imagine that. You mean quality, safety, and reliability are two tiers from the President of the United States?"

"He was showing that you don't get quality by accident, you have to care about it, you have to manage it into the system," Berwick notes. Guy Cohen talked at length about the organization chart and the process NASA used. Berwick was struck by NASA's transparent culture, a culture that encouraged people to come forward with mistakes—that focused on finding defects and fixing the process that allowed the mistakes to occur. "Guy was actually showing me the real stuff, and my God, they got to the moon!"

NASA's relationship with subcontractors was emblematic of their approach. While some companies sought to squeeze subcontractors purely on price, NASA sought to form a partnership with their subcontractors, negotiating fair prices in return for ongoing relationships, dependability, and superb quality. Cohen said that NASA had direct personal relationships with seventh subcontractors, that is, the subs of subs of subs, and so forth. He noted that NASA officials would go to those subcontractors with a message: "That rocket has in it a pump which has a whirring thing, which has a blade, which has metal . . . and that little bit of metal is going to be a vane, which is going to go into a blade, which is going on a gyroscope, which is going to be in a guidance system, which is going to go in the top part of the rocket, and there is a man sitting in the seat whose life depends on what you do."

Cohen said to Berwick: "It's very, very important to be able to connect the meaning of their work to their work." "That was really interesting," says Berwick, who was struck by the power of Cohen's statement. "Here's medicine full of meaning and who had ever said that?"

Then Guy Cohen told Berwick a story he has never forgotten, one that is emblazoned onto his memory because Berwick believes it speaks volumes about the way health care *should* work. It was a story about a missing bolt: a single bolt in a liquid oxygen tank on a Titan rocket. Cohen explained that on the eve of a launch a worker in protective gear was lowered into the tank to make repairs and retrieve two bolts, but he came out with only one. The worker said he believed there had been only one bolt inside the tank. This was crucial; a loose bolt inside the tank held the potential for disaster. They had to get this right. The team flashed powerful beams down into the tank. "No bolt was there, they all agreed, and, reassured, they closed the hatch again. Launch was the next morning."

But one of Guy's team members, a junior quality control officer named Gerry Gonsalves, was troubled by the fact that only one bolt had been retrieved. Berwick would later recount:

> Gerry had been sent to the assembly plant in Denver to act as the "missile chaperone" for the next Titan to be sent to Florida for launch. In the wee hours of the morning, he crawled from his bed and drove to a storage plant where there happened to be a spare, identical twin of the liquid oxygen tank he had inspected on the launch pad. On hands and knees, with a spare bolt and some transparent tape, Gerry crawled in and out of the tank seeing if just possibly he could fix the loose bolt into a location that was invisible from the open hatch. He found two such locations.

At 2:00 A.M., he awoke Guy Cohen at home to tell him of the hazard. "We could have missed the bolt," Gerry told Guy. "We might have screwed up."

Guy scrubbed the launch. At 8:00 the next morning, instead of watching a rocket lift off, the team reassembled on the launch pad. Again they lowered the man into the tank. It took him thirty seconds to find the loose bolt, precisely in one of the two spots that Gerry Gonsalves had identified the night before.

"What did NASA do?" Berwick asked Guy, knowing that in health care there would have been recriminations.

"We gold-plated the bolt," said Guy, "and made a tie clip out of it for Gerry. The quality control director presented an award the day that Titan was finally launched—and hit its target. It was more important to reward, not censure, to make certain that accurate information would flow freely and not be covered up."

For Berwick, this was an immensely powerful story: "I thought of my own world of malpractice suits, quality assurance investigations, performance reviews . . . and then I thought of the world Guy Cohen was describing with that story—a world of openness, involvement, celebration, and dedication to excellence."

Berwick then traveled to New Jersey to visit Bell Laboratories, renowned for fanatical attention to quality detail. He was particularly impressed by one employee who told Berwick about his work on a switching system for a 3,000-mile-long, fiber-optic undersea cable that runs across the Atlantic. Since light attenuates as it travels, it has to be "boosted," or re-amplified, at regular intervals. Though Bell designed the booster to last a hundred years, there's also a remote-controlled backup booster in case of failure. "To rotate it requires a little motor that moves it into place," Berwick remembers. "So here's a motor that has to work *once*, maybe, in the next hundred years in order to save a billion-dollar cable. . . . And they do it! And I'm thinking, 'We can't get Mrs. Jones her penicillin at the right time of day.' They're talking about failure, maybe, in one switch, maybe, eighty-eight years from now and *they can do it.*"

While Don Berwick continued searching outside health care for quality ideas, another quality pioneer, Paul Batalden, MD, had embarked on a similar path. Batalden was already years ahead of Berwick. By the time Berwick met with NASA and Bell Labs, Batalden had been exploring the world of industrial quality for four years; indeed, he had written about quality as early as 1977.

Batalden grew up in Minneapolis, where he attended Augsburg College and the University of Minnesota Medical School. With a slim build, well-trimmed beard, and fair, Scandinavian complexion, he appeared younger than he was. Batalden had a quick laugh and easy manner; he was eminently approachable and something of a mad genius. He read philosophy voraciously, Germans in particular.

After medical school, his desire to pursue a deeper understanding of medical science led him to the National Institutes of Health (NIH), the sprawling federal agency that conducts and supports a wide array of scientific research. He worked as a clinical associate in the NIH Acute Leukemia Service for Children in Bethesda, Maryland, with a focus on specialized academic pediatric gastroenterology. NIH was an eye-opener for Batalden. Though it was one of the most prestigious medical centers in the world, from Batalden's perspective (and that of other young doctors) it suffered real and obvious deficiencies. As they struggled to care for critically ill children, consults would go unanswered. "Lab results came back to us in mountains of paperwork that we had to sift through to find the critical data meaning it was easy to miss important stuff," he recalls. "I was quite frustrated about the quality of patient care."

Hoping to expand his horizons, Batalden left NIH. In 1969, at age twenty-seven, he accepted a position as medical director of the Job Corps, an education and vocational training program for young Americans. When he was twenty-nine, he ascended to a position as assistant surgeon general in the U.S. Public Health Service as director of the Community Health Services.

In 1975, Batalden returned to his hometown of Minneapolis, where he continued his work on health care quality and health policy as quality assurance project director at InterStudy, a Minneapolis-based health policy group instrumental in developing the federal HMO policy and program. At the same time, Batalden worked as a pediatrician caring for the children of about 1,000 families. If that wasn't enough, he soon became chief operating officer of Park Nicollet Medical Center—all this as he continued to see patients. This was a time of cutting-edge research and study for Batalden, a time filled with new ideas about health policy generally and quality in particular. Batalden and his colleagues developed a model of quality improvement (and subsequently wrote a book about it: *Quality Assurance in Ambulatory Care*). Like Berwick's efforts at HCHP, Batalden and his colleagues culled a small sample of patients and then aggregated their responses. Says Batalden:

> For many doctors it was the first time they received "unvarnished" feedback. In this material, ob-gyn doctors were not told how much their patients loved them—they were told how egocentric they were in having scheduling methods that made it nearly impossible for their patients to see them. They were told how maddening it was to have to book an appointment nearly one year ahead. An ophthalmologist was told by a patient that the patient couldn't understand how such a smart man could do such a stupid thing as smoke. . . . Another doctor learned that his patients thought he always seemed angry. .

No one threw anything at Paul Batalden, but that did not mean the doctors liked what they were hearing. A physician approached Batalden one day and said: "I'd love your job—you go around putting a monkey on another person's back."

"No, actually," Batalden replied. "My job is to go around and give the news that you have a monkey on your back and I'd love to help get it off."

Batalden made one of his more important discoveries on the morning of Sunday, May 10, 1981, when he read an article in the *New York Times* about a man named W. Edwards Deming. Batalden had never heard of him, but Deming was as famous among Japanese business people as he was anonymous in the United States; indeed, he was none other than the management guru whose ideas had helped revive Japan in the postwar years. The article portrayed Deming as a "sprightly octogenarian" and "an unlikely looking celebrity, this 80-year-old man with thick glasses perched on his beak-like nose." Yet the article ordained Deming as "the high prophet of quality control" and nothing less than "an unadulterated superstar."

"We're in a new economic age," the *Times* quoted Deming. "We cannot tolerate poor quality work anymore. *We're in an age when one defect in 5,000 is too many* [emphasis added]."

With an undergraduate degree from the University of Wyoming and a PhD in mathematical physics from Yale, Deming worked for the U.S. Census Bureau. In 1946, he became an independent consultant preaching a unique gospel of quality improvement to companies and organizations (while in his spare time studying music theory, composing two masses, and playing a variety of instruments).

His greatest success came in Japan in the 1950s. Using Deming's approach to quality improvement, Japanese manufacturers (electronic, automotive, and others) dramatically increased quality, productivity, and profitability. Before Deming's methods were adopted, Japanese goods were notoriously poorly made, yet not long after the adoption of Deming's approach Japanese manufacturing became a model for the world. According to the *Times* article, Deming was so revered in Japan that the Japanese created the Deming Prize for achievement in product quality.

Deming preached that it was the responsibility of senior company executives to install a continuous quality system that would yield the finest possible products and services. When he was hired to consult with a company, he would insist that senior management attend his sessions. At one meeting in Michigan, the CEO left to take a phone call and, when he did so, Deming sat down and fell silent. Dozens of employees sat in awkward silence until it was made abundantly clear that Deming had no intention of continuing until the CEO returned to the room.

As he read the *Times* that morning, Paul Batalden felt a stirring sense of intellectual excitement. He was particularly drawn to the portion of the article in which Deming stressed that most quality problems result not from bad workers but from faulty systems. Deming believed that properly managed organizations would inevitably increase quality and reduce costs. This view struck some business people as Pollyannaish. Conventional wisdom held that quality was expensive; quality meant more workers, more inspection, more expensive equipment. But that was all wrong, Deming said. Defective products rolling off assembly lines or factory floors required time, effort, and money, and discovering that they were defective after the fact meant much wasted time, effort, and money. Instead, Deming preached building quality into the manufacturing process rather than leaving it until the end. "In effect, a company is paying workers to make defects and then to correct them. Quality comes not from inspection but from improvement in the process."

Conventional wisdom viewed manufacturing as a series of bits and pieces. Assemble this piece, attach it to that, connect it to something else. But Deming saw it as a seamless process. Workers on the front lines were the key, he said. It was the workers, not management, who knew what was wrong with the process or system. Deming said that managers needed to get down on the factory floor and learn from their workers. If managers gained the knowledge of workers, they would be equipped to construct a manufacturing process that excluded defects, avoided waste, and allowed for continuous improvement.

After reading the *Times* article, Batalden telephoned Deming and asked how he could learn more. Deming suggested that Batalden attend one of his four-day seminars, so Batalden flew to Atlanta for Deming's seminar of December 7–10, 1981. The course ("Japanese

Methods for Productivity and Quality") was based on Deming's book *Quality, Productivity and Competitive Position*. Batalden and a physician colleague traveled to the session uncertain what to expect, generally assuming that Deming would elaborate on the issues raised in the *Times* article. Initially, Deming's course disappointed Batalden. The conditions were unpleasant: The room was packed with engineers puffing on cigarettes, a cloud of smoke hung over the audience as Deming stood on the stage, the sound system screeching feedback, and read aloud from his book in a ponderous, droning style.

There was something unusual, even odd about Deming. He was tall with an elongated head, almost bullet-shaped, with glasses and a severe gaze. He came across as a serious man who gave no hint of frivolity, and he possessed a clipped manner. Worst of all, from what Batalden could follow, Deming seemed to be talking about, of all things, ball bearings. Puzzled by what was happening, Batalden approached Deming during a break and asked whether he was free for dinner. Deming told Batalden he allowed one hour for dinner and that if Batalden wanted to join him for those sixty minutes he would be welcome. "He was eighty-one years old and by dinner time he had lectured for nine hours and he budgets one hour for dinner," Batalden says. "There was a lot of energy there, something really driving him."

By the time dinner was through, Batalden had a different take on Deming. "As we talked, he shared his views about the way the health care system worked, what he observed, etc. I realized he was used to 'seeing things' with different lenses. I went back to the lectures. . . . I saw that he was not really talking about manufacturing . . . it was a theory of work, which conceptualized the continual improvement of quality as intrinsic to the work itself."

Batalden realized that Deming saw whole systems at work. "He didn't see a doctor and then a nurse and then a patient—he saw them as interdependent elements of a system and he looked for how that system could work better." The essence of the four-day seminar centered on Deming's "Fourteen Points," which contained the heart of his thinking. In essence, an organization that applied and integrated the fourteen points would increase efficiency, productivity, and quality. Among the more cogent points presented at the session Batalden attended were:

- Create and communicate to all employees a statement of the aims and purposes of the company.
- Build quality into a product throughout production.
- End the practice of awarding business on the basis of price tag alone; instead, try a long-term relationship based on established loyalty and trust.
- Work to constantly improve quality and productivity.
- Institute on-the-job training.
- Drive out fear; create trust.
- Strive to reduce intradepartmental conflicts.
- Remove barriers that rob people of pride of workmanship.
- Include everyone in the company to accomplish the transformation.

The approach embodied in the fourteen points was just what health care needed, thought Batalden. By the time the four-day session was over, Batalden felt the excitement that comes with a new discovery. He was so enthusiastic that on the airplane back to Minneapolis he feverishly worked to capture the ideas and nuances of Deming's thinking so it would apply to health care. Batalden was now so convinced that he had discovered a way for health care to increase quality that he was in a state of uber-production; indeed, he completed a draft of the translation before the jet touched down in Minneapolis. He let it sit on his desk for a few days, reviewed it, and decided it was precisely what he wanted to say—then he sent it off to Deming.

Several weeks later, Batalden received a phone call from Deming, who was writing a new book and wanted to use Batalden's translation nearly verbatim. This was extraordinary: Deming, a curmudgeon's curmudgeon, was paying Batalden the highest possible compliment, that he had got Deming's principles almost exactly right (Deming had a few changes, of course); so right, in fact, that he wanted them for his own book. Naturally, Batalden granted permission for the use of his translation and it appeared in Deming's book *Out of the Crisis*. Batalden's version was quite a bit longer than Deming's original fourteen points, and key sections enunciated his vision for quality in health care.

"We can no longer live with commonly accepted levels of mistakes," Batalden wrote. This was a revolutionary statement in health care and Paul Batalden knew it. The year was 1981, and Batalden's translation of the Deming approach was so fundamentally sound that it would serve as the foundation for the new quality movement a quarter century later. Why was Batalden's declaration such a crucial moment? Until then, and the assumption is still common throughout medicine, the general belief was that mistakes were an integral and unavoidable by-product of health care; that they had always happened, would always happen, and there was nothing much anyone could do about it. Mistakes by clinicians were often camouflaged as "complications." All patients understood that complications were possible—even when clinicians were doing their best—and patients accepted that term. Through the years, however, the term has evolved to become a catch-all not only for unavoidable or unexpected difficulty in a case but also for excusing or covering up preventable medical errors.

Deming, of course, believed systems could be devised to virtually eliminate "complications." Systems had been devised to all but eliminate defects in manufacturing, but in health care no one had ever even tried, and certainly not on a broad and sustained basis. Batalden addressed inspection versus built-in quality, a key aspect of the Deming approach: "Inspection is not the answer. Inspection is too late and is unreliable. Inspection does not produce quality."

While Paul Batalden is deeply cerebral, he is also very much a man of action. Once he absorbed the Deming approach he went right to work to apply those principles in a real health care setting. He convinced Tommy Frist, CEO of the Healthcare Corporation of America (HCA), to fund a quality resource group within HCA, which at the time consisted of 390 hospitals in forty-seven states and eight foreign countries—an extraordinary laboratory for Batalden's quality work. Frist agreed, and Batalden established basic quality improvement courses that he and his team taught to thousands of HCA employees as a way of spreading the quality gospel. Though HCA is a for-profit company, Batalden insisted, and Frist agreed, that any quality improvement they discovered internally would be shared with the health care world at large. "Quality is not a proprietary item in health care," Batalden said.

Batalden is a modest man, but he did not conceal his ambitions at the time. When asked by his good friend and colleague Gene Nelson what he was trying to accomplish at HCA, Batalden replied: "I just want to change the way we think about health care in the United States."

For some years, Paul Batalden and Don Berwick had been working on their own. But when they finally met, it created the core of a leadership team that would play a critical role in leading the new quality movement for decades to come. Berwick recalls that they first encountered one another at a conference in Boston in the mid-1980s. They talked a good deal that day, and it was clear they shared a mission. Since it was pouring that evening in the city, Berwick gave Batalden a lift to his hotel. By the time they had finished their discussions for the day, Batalden had invited Berwick to Nashville to speak to some of his colleagues at HCA.

From the very first there was a sense of connection between them, a sense that their thinking and visions were aligned. In fact, there were striking parallels between the two men. Just a few years apart in age, both men were unusually articulate, and both possessed an air of easy charisma that attracted others to their ideas and leadership. They had extraordinarily agile minds coupled with an energetic and persistent sense of curiosity and a penchant for tackling difficult issues. During their early discussions, Batalden gently recommended that Berwick study Deming. Berwick took up Batalden's suggestion and signed up for a Deming seminar in Washington, D.C., in 1986. It would prove to be one of the more bizarre, yet meaningful, experiences of Berwick's career. As he listened to Deming's unique style of lecturing, he experienced a mounting sense of annoyance:

> It was very visceral [Berwick recalls]. I was sweating, I couldn't sit. . . . I was just in the wrong place. It was a roomful of industry people, and these people from chemical industries, lumber, and here I was, a doctor . . . and I just thought, "Where the hell am I?" And then this guy was droning on and on and on, ". . . *and on page 267 you will find. . . .*" Very monotonic teaching. . . . "Do you have constancy of purpose for improvement?" That's his famous first point. . . . "Do you have constancy of purpose for improvement?" . . . I thought it was drivel. I thought, "What is this constancy of purpose for improvement?" It sounded so foreign, so different to me. A lot of it was from manufacturing. So here I was, a doctor . . . and he's talking about manufacturing.

Berwick grew so agitated that he actually got up, left the room, caught a taxi to the airport, and flew back to Boston. He was in an emotional state, a state of great agitation, but he did not know why. At home that night he became deeply unsettled.

"I felt *so* uncomfortable. I just felt this was terrible. . . . At the time I thought it was his teaching style—he droned on for hours. I came home that night, went to bed and woke up about 2:00 in the morning, sweating." It was then that the revelation struck him: *"Everything Deming was saying was right."* Berwick had invested so much in the inspection process, in examining what had happened after the fact, and now it was clear to him that Deming was saying it was all wrong; that it was crap, garbage, a waste of time. He realized that the physician who had thrown the report at him was right and he was wrong. He had been an inspector rather than a promoter of quality. Deming was saying that after-the-fact inspection was a waste and the improvement throughout the process was what really yielded quality results. Says Berwick:

> At the Harvard Plan I had built an extremely strong inspection apparatus. I could produce reports on anything. Tables and graphs showing how 83 percent of the patients are waiting thirty minutes or more, whatever, anything you want. I had spent years, five years of my career packaging that stuff, reporting it to management, reporting it to the work force, experiencing anger and push back, with not much progress. I thought it was about motivation and . . . just kind of like I wasn't yelling loud enough and I needed to wake these people up or whatever any inspector who cares about what they're doing, is doing.

Now here was Deming explaining a quality management system based on statistics, on science—on the idea of continuous quality improvement—the idea of building quality into the process and the product rather than simply creating products, then inspecting them after the fact and tossing out the bad apples. "And that was the sweat in the middle of the night . . . just 'Oh, my God, I'm doing this wrong.'"

The next morning, with his wife thinking he had lost his marbles, Berwick rushed to catch a plane back to Washington to attend the rest of the seminar. Berwick looked forward to meeting Deming at a dinner with several others attending the seminar. That night at the Cosmos Club, an oasis for lofty achievers in science and the arts housed in a striking French Renaissance building in northwest Washington, Berwick was still somewhat agitated. He was struggling with the notion that Deming's discussions of industrial quality improvement might have bearing on health care. At one point during dinner, Berwick asked Deming directly whether his methods would work in health care. But Edwards Deming turned away from Berwick, ignoring his question.

Looking back, Berwick realizes that Deming didn't have anything to tell him. "My questions were too far away from where he was," says Berwick. "I would have to learn a lot more to be able to have a conversation with him. . . . He was intolerant of me. I asked him a couple of questions, and I'm sure right away he knew that I hadn't really read his book yet. He wasn't going to spend his time with a novice. . . . 'Call me when you've actually studied it a little bit' is what he really wanted to say."

As rocky as his introduction to Deming had been, however, Berwick soon became a convert. Berwick read a great deal by and about Deming, and he discussed his approach with Paul Batalden at some length. Like Batalden, Berwick arrived at the conviction that Deming's approach to quality could make a serious impact on health care. By October 1987, Berwick was drawing from Deming's work in testimony Berwick delivered to the U.S. House Subcommittee on Health and the Environment of the Energy and Commerce Committee.

"More than ever before," Berwick testified, "there is an uneasiness about quality in American health care today." He continued that "quality problems in industrial settings tend to be systems problems.

The opportunities for improvement of quality lie in improved design of systems, and I believe that this is also true of health care systems."

Decades later, this has become accepted wisdom, but at the time, Berwick and Batalden were unique in their vision.

Although much of Berwick's work in the new quality movement was necessarily cerebral and theoretical, he also learned from personal experiences. In a speech at the Sixth Annual National Forum on Quality Improvement in Health Care organized by IHI in December 1994, Berwick recounted the story of what happened to his father earlier that year. Berwick's father fell and broke his hip and was taken by ambulance to the hospital. The senior Dr. Berwick also suffered from Parkinson's disease and mild dementia at the time. Don Berwick's brother, who lived much closer to the hospital than Don, rushed to the hospital to meet their father at the emergency room. When he arrived at the hospital and asked for their father, he was told that he was not there. "Panicked phone calls followed as my brother searched anxiously for our father, until finally someone told him that our father was there after all and was about to be wheeled to the operating room," Berwick says. His father's recovery did not go well. Within a week his right heel developed a deep pressure ulcer that prevented him from walking, a key aspect of rehabilitation.

Berwick and his brother found the best rehab facility in the area and placed their father there:

> I visited him there on the morning after his admission [wrote Berwick]. He was lying stuporous in the bed, on his back, with his ulcerated heel pressing into the sheets. His mouth was hanging open and his eyes were rolled back into his head. I asked the nurse for an explanation. "We sedated him," she said. "He was combative. He hit a staff member." For ten years he has had severe Parkinson's disease, and for most of that time he has been unable to extend his own arm voluntarily,

much less throw a [punch]. My father had undoubtedly been angry, yes. But a punch—no. I demanded that the sedation be stopped.

Berwick also discovered that his father's Parkinson's medication, meticulously adjusted for two years by his physician at home, had been stopped without explanation when he was admitted to the rehabilitation facility. For two weeks, the senior Dr. Berwick was wracked with spasms and decreased mobility.

"When my brothers and I asked that our father be placed in a wheelchair whenever possible, the weekend shift of nurses told us that no wheelchairs could be found. They asked that we bring in his rickety old wheelchair from home. They eventually did find a wheelchair, but it was missing the footrest plate that would have protected his injured heel from bruising," Berwick recounts.

The combination of his father's experience and Deming's teachings served as a powerful lesson for Berwick. The two experiences were, in a way, sources of fuel that propelled Berwick forward. Through Deming, Berwick's store of intellectual knowledge expanded greatly. And through his father's experience, Berwick's visceral understanding of the dysfunctional nature of the system was seared into his mind. Don Berwick wasn't exactly sure where to go next, but he knew that he had somehow to combine the two—the Deming knowledge and the real-life experience—if he was to succeed in advancing the cause.

2

The Birth of IHI

———— ∞∞∞ ————

"You're the MD and you do a beautiful diagnosis. But what if blood is drawn from the wrong patient? What if you cannot read the x-ray? What if the pharmacist doesn't put the right thing in the bottle? We're talking about managing a system!"

In the coming years, Berwick immersed himself in studying the rich field of industrial quality, delving not only into Deming but also reading the work of Walter Shewhart, PhD, a physicist, statistician, and engineer who headed quality at Bell Labs early in the twentieth century. Shewhart saw that after-the-fact inspection wasted time and money and produced inferior results. Shewhart was the visionary who saw that quality resulted from a well-designed process—revolutionary thinking nearly a century ago. Berwick studied other giants in the field as well, including Joseph Juran, a Romanian-born industrial engineer, and Ichiro Ishikawa, an important contributor to Japanese quality improvement. Berwick could see that rigorous work by engineers and statisticians had created a solid foundation for modern quality management based on statistical evidence.

Although Berwick was a forceful and articulate advocate for these theories, convincing highly skeptical health care stakeholders that industrial quality techniques would work in health care was a challenge. He needed proof, and the opportunity came with an idea from Blanton Godfrey, the head of Bell Labs Quality Theory and Technology Department. He suggested a simple solution: Put the industrial techniques to the test in a demonstration project. Godfrey enjoyed credibility in the field. Berwick had read Godfrey's book *Modern Methods for Quality Control and Improvement* (coauthored with Harrison M. Wadsworth and Kenneth S. Stephens), a classic treatise on quality. At 700-plus pages, with dense, industrial, engineering, and statistical language, the book was not for the faint of heart, yet Berwick devoured it.

With a grant from the Hartford Foundation, Berwick and Godfrey enlisted the participants. Berwick signed on twenty-one blue-chip hospitals, group practices, and HMOs, ranging from Massachusetts General to Kaiser Permanente, from Johns Hopkins to the University of Michigan. And Godfrey brought in an equally impressive group of quality mentors ranging from Ford to Xerox, from AT&T to NASA. They set an aggressive timeline: The projects would commence in September 1987 with phase one completion by June 1988.

Thus was born the National Demonstration Project on Quality Improvement in Health Care, more commonly known as the National Demonstration Project (NDP). The NDP process was simple: Teams consisting of quality experts from industry and clinicians as well as administrators from the hospital would select a problem to work on—Children's Hospital in Boston, for example, sought to shorten the transport time of critically ill infants from remote hospitals—then diagnose the problem by gathering information on the process to get at its root cause. The teams would work toward a remedy, testing various options along the way, all the while monitoring performance and making adjustments in the attempt to answer one question: Can the tools of modern quality improvement, with which other industries have achieved breakthroughs in performance, help in health care as well?

The projects themselves tackled a wide variety of problems. Administrative errors in Medicare billing were causing Massachusetts General Hospital to lose millions of dollars annually; administrators at Park Nicollet Medical Center in Minnesota were overwhelmed with telephone calls from patients in the family practice unit; several hospitals in Michigan, North Carolina, and Massachusetts experienced lengthy discharge delays that, in turn, prevented rooms from becoming available to new patients in a timely manner; and at Harvard Community Health Plan (HCHP) the use of ultrasonography in pregnant women varied significantly.

Industry experts found their health care counterparts largely ignorant of quality improvement tools and techniques, but they also found that health care people were bright, quick learners. Through Berwick, Godfrey, and Paul E. Plsek, a consultant hired by Godfrey and Berwick, the teams learned various quality improvement techniques. Virtually all the teams started their work with a common industrial quality improvement tool known as a process flow diagram, a simple yet revealing graphic representation of the steps in the process surrounding the problem. The tool allowed teams to see—many for the first time—exactly what the process was, and, quite often, seeing the process enabled teams to pinpoint the source of the problem. As Berwick and his colleagues later observed, the teams would apply a tool, see the data clearly, and respond: "So *that's* why the hospital records aren't getting into the patient's regular files" and "So *that's* why the operating room gets backed up every day."

After nine months, the teams reported on their work. Most had progressed on an administrative or business process. The Kaiser-Permanente project, for example, focused on figuring out how to get emergency department clinical data from the ER to various Kaiser satellite locations in different towns. Too often, after patients had been seen in the ER, they would go for follow-up care and their records would still be back at the ER, miles away, or in transit. This was immensely frustrating to doctors, who could not properly treat a patient without an accurate record. Since the absence of a record subjected doctors to an increased risk of making an error in treatment, physicians frequently refused to treat a patient until the record arrived. The time taken to track down and get the record to the site meant significant delays and wasted time for doctors and patients.

The Kaiser project used rudimentary quality improvement tools, including process flow diagrams, and discovered that the actual process for moving records from the ER to the satellite facilities was surprisingly different from what they had originally thought. This important revelation showed that physicians and administrators were not aware of how things *actually* worked at their own facility.

When the team learned how chaotic the existing process was, it was relatively simple to fashion a more orderly system that sent patient records from the ER to satellite offices where patients would be seen for follow-ups. With the new process, ten times as many records arrived at the right places than before. In one location, the rate of success of getting the right record to the correct location rose from 23 to 70 percent. What did this mean in terms of quality? It meant that doctors not only had the information they needed at the time of examination but also a better chance of selecting the right treatment; it meant that doctors weren't wasting their time waiting for stray records. It was, in other words, a meaningful change that helped support the delivery of quality care.

Similar successes were achieved in numerous NDP projects, yet the hole in NDP was its focus on administrative rather than clinical improvements. The team from Butterworth Hospital in Grand Rapids did, in fact, tackle an important clinical issue—improving respiratory care—and the Boston Children's Hospital group worked on improving the transport speed of critically ill infants. Most of the NDP participants, however, "stayed on the comfortable fringes," as Berwick put it, "working on problems in medical organizations that more directly resembled quality problems in other industries." This approach, as Berwick observed, meant that the teams did not have to battle clinicians over turf or clinical procedures.

During the course of NDP, teams generally found it difficult to persuade doctors to join them; some said they were too busy while others were skeptical that quality approaches from other industries had a place in health care. At this stage in the history of the new quality movement, of course, only a handful of doctors had been introduced to the notion that industrial quality might apply to clinical issues, and their reactions were all but uniform: *There's no assembly line in health care. We're not making cars, we're dealing with human beings and every patient is different.*

It was clear to Berwick that the new quality movement was going nowhere without doctors. The cultural reality in hospitals was that physicians ruled, and there was little tolerance for reforms that in any way were perceived as impinging on their clout or relationships with patients. As a practicing physician seeing patients one day a week, Berwick well understood this mentality, and he knew firsthand the sacrosanct nature of the doctor-patient relationship. But he also knew that much of what actually happened in health care took place outside that relationship; he also believed that much of health care could be streamlined and made safer and more efficient with the application of quality systems. Berwick and his colleagues later wrote:

[B]arriers to physician involvement may turn out to be the most important single issue impeding the success of quality improvement in medical care. Industrial quality relied on measurement and standardization of practices[,] and doctors were generally deeply suspicious of both—measurement because of its association with policing activities; physicians are suspicious that measurement allegedly for improvement may instead be used for judgment and surveillance.

Physicians are suspicious of standardization because many doctors share the belief that medicine is an art. The common reaction to standardization of procedures by doctors was to deride it as "cookbook medicine."

Batalden also saw doctors as formidable obstacles. He believed that doctors often tended to be "in love with what they were doing and to suggest that these smart people should do something different was an affront." All their adult lives, says Batalden, doctors have been taught to take individual responsibility for patients: "We were taught that if you worked and studied hard enough things wouldn't go wrong. This notion of individual responsibility is so deeply ingrained in our thinking that the idea of a *system* of care in which you worked was never given a seat at the table."

There were other impediments to the growth of the new quality movement, of course. Most social movements rode a popular uprising to prominence, but in health care there had been little in the way of a grassroots movement for quality. If patients weren't complaining, reasoned doctors and hospital leaders, why change? The movement towards quality was also stymied by the health care payment system, which compensated doctors and hospitals for procedures rather than for outcomes. As long as doctors and hospitals are paid for volume of procedures rather than for quality of outcomes they have little incentive to change. Providers were paid for exams and tests, but very rarely for quality; indeed, they were often paid more for lack of quality. To Berwick and Batalden at that moment, their most vehement opponents were their own colleagues.

Blan Godfrey was also astonished by the absence of process thinking in health care, especially on the part of MDs. As he recalls:

> That was the thing that blew my mind. I had not understood until then that they did not work across departments. Within their own boundaries they worked well but they didn't work well across boundaries. They didn't understand how the other pieces worked. I'd say to them, "You're the MD—the perfect person for this case and you do a beautiful diagnosis. But what if blood is drawn from the wrong patient? What if you cannot read the x-ray? What if the x-ray is not from your patient? What if the pharmacist doesn't put the right thing in the bottle? What we're talking about is managing the *system*—putting pieces together so that this very complicated thing called health care works. And you're just one tiny little piece in the whole process.

Going forward, Berwick and others in the movement would have to figure out ways to engage more doctors in the quality effort. In the meantime, they focused on what NDP had accomplished—small yet important discoveries. For one thing, the quality tools common in industry had proved easily adaptable to health care, and some of the experiments yielded positive results. NDP generated a series of quality improvement courses, created by Berwick, Batalden, Blan Godfrey, and others, that were drawn largely from the curriculum Batalden had built at the Healthcare Corporation of America (HCA). In the years to come, the courses would be taught to thousands of health care workers throughout the country.

In some ways, the most significant NDP achievement was the introduction of people in health care to industrial quality techniques; the very fact that a conversation had been started between industry and health care was a breakthrough. Berwick viewed this coming to-gether as creating "a very interesting community of insight." NDP had fostered a group of like-minded people in health care who could plainly see that although the experiments were far from conclusive there were considerable possibilities in bringing tools from industry to a health care setting.

Though NDP was hardly perfect, Berwick was energized by the experience. He wrote an article—"Continuous Improvement as an Ideal in Health Care"—published in the *New England Journal of Medicine* in 1989 and would be reprinted and quoted for years to come. It was Berwick's vision comparing how the health care system actually worked with how it might work.

IMAGINE two assembly lines, monitored by two foremen.

Foreman 1 walks the line, watching carefully. "I can see you all," he warns. "I have the means to measure your work, and I will do so. I will find those among you who are unprepared or unwilling to do your jobs, and when I do there will be consequences. . . . [Y]ou can be replaced."

Foreman 2 walks a different line, and he too watches. "I am here to help you if I can," he says. "We are in this together for the long haul. You and I have a common interest in a job well done. I know that most of you are trying very hard, but sometimes things can go wrong. My job is to notice opportunities for improvement—skills that could be shared, lessons from the past, or experiments to try together—and to give you the means to do your work even better than you do now."

Which line works better? Which is more likely to do the job well in the long run? Where would you rather work?

The theory used by Foreman 1 relies on inspection to improve quality. We may call it the Theory of Bad Apples, because those who subscribe to it believe that quality is best achieved by discovering bad apples and removing them from the lot.

The view is that problems of quality are caused by poor intentions. The Bad Apple is to blame. The cause of trouble is people—their venality, incompetence, or insufficient caution.

Berwick argued that the bad apple theory not only did not work but had slowed American industry even as the Japanese sprinted ahead on the strength of continuous quality improvement. He noted that American companies had even been forced to concede defeat to the Japanese in production of videocassette recorders and CD players ("Xerox engineers visiting Japan in 1979 found copiers being produced at half the cost of those manufactured at Xerox's facilities, with . . . 1/30 the number of defects").

The "community of insight" Berwick described as coming together around the National Demonstration Project needed to figure out the next steps. Yes, the potential was great, the possibilities exciting, but what next? Gene Nelson, a colleague of Batalden's was in the thick of the new quality movement. Nelson had earned his MA at Yale and PhD at Harvard and had studied deeply in the area of quality measurement both at RAND and HCA, where he had been mentored by Batalden. Nelson's expertise was the relatively new academic discipline of measuring quality in health care. He had collaborated on one of the most important quantitative studies: the RAND Medical Outcomes Study. Nelson's mantra: "To define quality you have to measure it." Nelson made a suggestion to Paul Batalden: *Let's get a small group of the true believers together—the revolutionaries—and meet on a regular basis and talk things through; see if we can learn from each other; see if we can figure out a way to advance the cause.*

Batalden liked the idea and thought about those who should be included. "We were all exploring this new way of thinking about quality in health care," says Batalden, who was also concerned about drawing the preemptive ire of people threatened by significant change. "We wanted to be free to explore what the ideas might mean and we wanted absolute trust. We came to the group mainly to learn; [we were] really interested in connecting our discoveries to each other."

In concert with Berwick, Paul Batalden and Gene Nelson selected just six other members carefully chosen for their intellect and passion for change. They were from Nashville and Boston, Detroit and Santa Monica, Madison and Chicago. There were nine in all, four MDs and five PhDs; experts in statistics, engineering, health care administration and regulation, social science, pediatrics, and psychometrics. The club's members included Paul Batalden, MD, then head of quality at HCA; James Roberts, MD, senior vice president of the Joint Commission; Dave Gustafson, PhD, professor of industrial engineering and preventive medicine at the University of Wisconsin–Madison, who had also worked as a consultant to Batalden at HCA; Vinod K. Sahney, PhD, senior vice president for strategy at Henry Ford Health System in Detroit, who also taught a course in operations management at the Harvard School of Public Health, where he met Berwick; James Schlosser, MD, MBA, had served as staff director of NDP; and John Ware, PhD, and Allyson Ross Davies, PhD, a husband-and-wife team from RAND, accomplished psychometricians and experts in the design of complex research projects such as using questionnaires to help define quality in health care.

Finally, there was Berwick, who was forty-two years old at the time and in the midst of the most unsettled period in his professional life. The Harvard Community Health Plan wanted a traditional measurement system, but Berwick had moved beyond such an approach and was reluctant to create one. This resulted in Berwick's reporting relationship being changed, a de facto demotion. Although he was "itchy" and wanted to leave, he was also anxious about departing a job that paid well and afforded ample benefits and security. His concern was reflected in an agenda item from a meeting in May 1991, where Berwick noted: "My future is crazy; an end will come in fall or winter." He had a conversation with his wife about leaving, but admitted that he was scared. Her response was emphatic: "You've got to do it."

It seemed only a matter of time before he was asked to leave, and so in 1989 Don Berwick decided it was time to move on. He had always had a secure job in health care, and leaving a comfortable position at one of the most innovative and prestigious HMOs in the country made him profoundly uneasy. Was he making a terrible mistake? Should he simply do what his superiors asked and find a way to work on his quality agenda in another forum?

The curse of innovators, of course, is a compulsion to follow their convictions, their *visions,* and Berwick was spurred by that compulsion. Berwick knew there was a better way for medicine, and he wanted to play a role in figuring it out. And so he left his administrative role at HCHP (though he continued to see patients one day a week, and stayed on as principal investigator on NDP). He also began doing consulting work on quality improvement to hospitals in Seattle, Pittsburgh, and elsewhere.

The consulting was fascinating, but Berwick's salvation during this period was the "community of insight" he found in Gene Nelson and Paul Batalden. Nicknamed the "Birthday Club" after their first meeting fell on Berwick's birthday, they met in airports for convenience sake—O'Hare, usually, but also Nashville and Boston. At their first session, in late 1988 while NDP was in progress, it quickly became clear that they all believed in a fundamentally heretical notion at the time: that the quality of care in America was deficient; that the system could be transformed; that transformation would bring about measurably better quality of care for millions of patients; and that countless lives could be saved.

Most American health care professionals at the time would have found this preposterous. Wasn't it true that we had the most advanced medical science research in the world, that we had the most innovative and brilliant surgeons, that people with the most difficult cases from throughout the world came to the United States for care, and that miracles were performed in major teaching hospitals across the length and breadth of the land every day? It was all true, of course, but Batalden, Berwick, and the others knew a very different story, a different truth that belied conventional wisdom. The truth involved preventable medical errors, systems that weren't really systems, wild inconsistency in quality of care, millions receiving care they didn't need, and millions more not receiving care that was known to be of great benefit.

How far out of the mainstream thinking of health care was the intellectual discourse at the Birthday Club? Gene Nelson said that if a hospital CEO had dropped in on a club meeting and listened for a while, the reaction would have been, "We don't know what you're talking about. We've got highly skilled physicians and nurses and it's their job to provide high quality care and they do. What might work for Motorola doesn't have relevance. We're not making high tech gizmos, we're taking care of patients."

While their ideas were controversial, the fact remained that through the courses they had begun, slowly but steadily, to build something of a following. NDP attracted some new supporters, as did Batalden's courses, which were taught at HCA and then NDP. The main course offerings included *An Introduction to Quality Improvement in Health Care* and *Methods and Tools of Quality Improvement*. They were taught at an executive conference center at Babson College in Wellesley, Massachusetts, not far from Boston. Typically, the courses ran from two and a half to three days and would be taught by Berwick, Batalden, Gustafson, and others. The students tended to be early adopters.

"In the initial wave it was mavericks, people who weren't generally sent there, but *chose* to go," recalls Berwick. "They found it somehow. . . . Maybe one third would be doctors, maybe 20 percent nurses and the rest quality improvement managers or people in charge of quality. A lot of them were the old style quality assurance officers, who now were starting to get the idea that something was new." Within a couple of years, the courses became so sought after that there was a waiting list, and about a hundred students attended each session. Inquiries came from throughout the world; over time, Berwick was invited to teach the course in a variety of countries, including Australia, Pakistan, Kenya, Israel, and Egypt.

Through all of this—NDP, the Birthday Club, his travels and speaking and writing—Don Berwick became something of an evangelist preaching the new quality gospel. He spoke often throughout the country and the world and wrote prolifically for a wide variety of publications, including the most prestigious medical journals. In early 1990, he had drafted an article he and Batalden planned but never found the time to finish. Berwick began in an arresting fashion:

Kim, age 3, lies asleep, waiting for a miracle. Outside her room the nurses on the night shift pad softly through the half-lighted corridors, stopping to count breaths, take pulses, or check the IV pumps.

In the morning, Kim will have her heart fixed. She will be medicated and wheeled to the operating suite. Machines will take on the functions of her body—breathing, circulating blood—while the surgeons place a small Kevlar patch over a hole within her heart, closing off a shunt between her ventricles that would, left open, slowly kill her.

Kim will be just fine if the decision to operate on her was correct. And if the surgeon is competent. And if that competent surgeon happens to be trained to deal with the particular anatomic wrinkle that Kim's heart contains. And if the blood-bank cross-matched her blood accurately, and delivered it to the right place. And if the blood gas analysis machine works properly and on time. And if the suture does not snap. And if the plastic tubing of the heart-lung machine does not suddenly spring loose. And if the recovery room nurses are aware of her allergy to penicillin. And if the oxygen and nitrogen lines in the anesthesia machine have not been reversed by mistake. And if the sterilizer temperature gauge is calibrated so that the instruments are sterile. And if the pharmacy does not mix up two labels. And if when the surgeon says urgently, "Clamp, right now," there is a clamp on the tray.

If all goes well—if ten thousand "ifs" go well—then Kim will sing her grandchildren to sleep some day. If not, she will be dead by noon tomorrow.

At a speech to a group of physicians at Park Nicollet in Minneapolis, Berwick described his source of inspiration. He said it came from a distant childhood memory, a time when he would be awakened from a deep sleep in the middle of the night by the sound of the telephone ringing next to his father's bed. After two rings—never more than that—Berwick would hear the water running in the bathroom briefly, and then the sound of his father's car starting. No matter what time, the senior Dr. Berwick would drive off to care for someone in need. That's what being a doctor was really all about: responding to those who needed you; going out in the middle of the night to cure, to comfort, to alleviate suffering. Every doctor understood this, and it was an understanding that bound physicians together like nothing else. In sharing this memory at Park Nicollet, Berwick sought to reassure the physicians that change in quality techniques would not disturb the essential mission or that doctor-patient relationship.

Referring to the audiences of doctors at Park Nicollet, Berwick says that "what we had in common was knowing what it's like to close the door and be in a room with a patient . . . [who] shares with you things they'll share with *no one else.*"

The other doctors in the Birthday Club understood this as well, but were at a point in their careers when their energies were devoted to healing patients by reforming the system. And central to the work of the club, perhaps its most important function, was working with and through Jim Roberts to effect policies at the Joint Commission. The commission is the most powerful accrediting body in American health care, an organization responsible for evaluating and accrediting some 15,000 health care organizations in the United States, including every major teaching hospital in the nation. Roberts was recruited to the Birthday Club by Paul Batalden, who considered him uniquely positioned, given his pivotal role at the Joint Commission, to impact quality of care. Since 1951, the commission had examined hospitals once every three years—examinations based upon a large number of standards set by the commission. The commission's reports granting or denying accreditation were always confidential.

The Birthday Club members saw the Joint Commission as an ideal pressure point, a place where a change in policies could impact every hospital in the country. If the Joint Commission promulgated a safety rule it became the medical law of the land. If the thoughts and ideas of the Birthday Club could work their way through Jim Roberts to the Commission and on to America's hospitals, the Birthday Club would have accomplished something meaningful. Dr. Jim Roberts quickly became a central member of the club cast. He brought a crucial perspective for he knew better than anyone else what it would take to align the Joint Commission with the new quality movement thinking.

"The Commission's standards reflected a way of thinking that was punitive," recalls Roberts. "If something happened somebody must have screwed up—Who was it and what are you going to do to him?" The assumption was that the problem was with people. The notion of process and system just wasn't part of the way we thought about quality.

For example, now we know . . . that if you give antibiotics an hour before surgery the chances of a postoperative infection are reduced substantially. The thinking was that if the antibiotic didn't get into the patient it was felt to be [the] surgeon's fault because he is the captain of the team. Now we understand that actually surgery is a very complicated *process* involving many people and all those individuals and things they do have to work together and there has to be a process that assures people get antibiotics an hour before surgery and in most of those steps—ordering, delivering, administering—the surgeon is not the person actually involved.

As he traveled to hospitals throughout the United States, Jim Roberts began to strike up discreet conversations with hospital administrators and physicians about quality. He would make the case that it was increasingly clear that health care was plagued by quality problems resulting not from incompetent people but from bad systems. Roberts believed that if he could help build a network of people who recognized the process problems, then new ideas, principally industrial quality techniques, might meet with greater acceptance. "It was very different saying this as opposed to saying, 'You have to do the Toyota Production System for industrial quality,' which people thought was odd or even offensive."

The Birthday Club was an intellectual oasis for Roberts. It provided him with a private setting where he could discuss ideas in confidence and get honest feedback on how to plot a course of change for the commission. Roberts knew that if the commission standards did not change the quality movement would make little real headway. Roberts was one of a number of senior Joint Commission officials who recognized the need for sweeping change. His boss, Dennis O'Leary, MD, president of the commission, was a visionary on the quality issue, and he had the support of the commission's board for change as well. Through the Birthday Club, Roberts established a network of connections to the vanguard of the new quality movement, which provided valuable feedback and advice about new Commission standards. "During the redesign of standards it was important to be able to touch base with those in the field who were in the forefront of the revolution in the way we thought about and did improvement in health care," Roberts says.

But none of the members of the club were delusional; all knew that the task of taking on quality in health care was monumental. Roberts defined the challenge in stark terms in a memo to his Birthday Club colleagues: "The vast majority of health care organizations have little, if any, knowledge of quality improvement and there is no health care organization that has a fully operational continual improvement program." Nonetheless, as time passed and the Birthday Club dug deeper into the issues, the group's sense of purpose strengthened. In time, there came over the group a powerful sense of confidence that they could effect change. Someone, probably Paul Batalden, even quoted Margaret Meade: "A small group of thoughtful people could change the world. Indeed, it's the only thing that ever has."

But revolutionary change would not come about if the Birthday Club continued to meet a few times a year in secret. To ignite real change, they realized, they needed another vehicle. There were options: teach more classes to more people about more subjects; create a department within a university, perhaps within a school of public health. Batalden insisted that the work would take at least twenty-five years and called for establishing an organization that would have the greatest possible chance to endure over time. Toward that end, in late 1991, the Birthday Club created the Institute for Healthcare

Improvement (IHI), an independent organization with the goal of transforming health care in the United States. It began with Berwick as CEO, Batalden as chairman of the board, and the other members of the Birthday Club among the board of directors. IHI took over responsibility for the courses that had come out of NDP. They were now IHI courses, and Berwick went to work expanding the course offerings and increasing the number of students.

Berwick loved the new organization. This was the work he truly wanted to do; this was the idea for which he had such an intense passion. Now he had his own operation in concert with a group of like-minded people. Now he was his own boss in effect (with Batalden as his chairman), and now he was free to do nothing but pursue the quality agenda in which he and his Birthday Club colleagues believed.

During the first year after the founding of IHI, it became clear that although the new quality revolution was quiet and largely unseen by mainstream medicine it was nonetheless growing and attracting passionately committed advocates. Berwick and members of the board continued teaching classes to overflowing crowds of doctors, nurses, administrators, and academics, winning over increasing numbers of converts.

That first year, Berwick and IHI organized the National Forum on Quality Improvement in Health Care. They invited people who had taken their courses as well as clinicians and quality people at hospitals throughout the country. The organization was in its infancy and very few people had ever heard of it, yet the response was impressive; the conference drew 1,600 people to Orlando for three days of work and discussion on quality. In his keynote speech, Berwick enthused: "How far we have come! A mere five or six years ago, the language of quality improvement, if not the ideas themselves, would have met with blank stares in most quarters of American health care."

But IHI had a problem. The group's classes drew impressive people from throughout the world, but what impact did they have on improving quality in the health care system? Vin Sahney, PhD, an IHI board member and quality expert from Henry Ford in Detroit, said that hospital administrators and clinicians would meet with IHI officials and enthusiastically agree that certain changes needed to be made and "then they would go home and a year would go by and nothing would happen." Berwick worried that they were engaged in "too much teaching and not enough action."

"We weren't making change happen," recalls Maureen Bisognano, the IHI chief operating officer. "There's an expression that it's 'a sin to send a changed man back to an unchanged organization,' but that's what was happening. Working through innovators—thousands had come to our classes and left motivated and excited—was not enough. They'd go back to organizations where nobody wanted to change."

Classes drew anywhere from fifty to a hundred participants, but never more than a few who had been sent by the organization's management. The overwhelming percentage had come on their own out of a desire to learn more about the quality movement. They learned about measurement and how data could drive quality. They learned about the science of improvement, drawn largely from the teachings of Deming and other industrial quality theorists.

But was this overly theoretical? Was it too academic to make a real impact? Tom Nolan, a PhD in statistics and a consultant to IHI, thought so, believing the organization should zero in more precisely on clinical improvement. Until then, most of the classes IHI offered taught people how to conduct improvement efforts within hospitals and other health care organizations. The teaching skills focused on Deming-like improvement processes. Nolan said that quality improvement was "derived from a combination of improvement knowledge," which IHI was teaching quite effectively, "coupled with subject matter knowledge"—the knowledge of specific clinical areas needing improvement. He argued that to be successful, IHI would have to help hospitals solve the real-world clinical problems they faced every day.

Nolan's prodding got the IHI leadership to think seriously about a new direction, and it came, as so often had been the case in the new quality movement, from the creative mind of Paul Batalden. His basic idea was simple: IHI would select a widespread clinical problem, convene leading experts on the topic, then invite hospitals and physician groups from throughout the country to join their learning session. Working under expert guidance, the group would define, for example, the current state of ICU care; then show the current example of the best ICU care available; and finally push toward defining a much better form of ICU care.

The program was dubbed the Breakthrough Series, and the notion was to start with the areas "ripe for improvement," as Berwick put it. Berwick said that research clearly showed that in many crucial areas of medicine, from Caesarian section surgery to diabetes care and from ICU practices to cardiac surgery, practices varied widely throughout the country, and many varied from what was known to be the best practice. Ideally, with experts and clinicians working together, a synergy would be created, thus triggering breakthrough improvements.

Bruce Flamm, MD, an expert on reducing Caesarian rates from Kaiser Permanente on the West Coast, agreed to help lead the Caesarian effort, as did Robert DeMott, MD, from Green Bay, Wisconsin. About thirty organizations joined in. The goal of the C-section project, according to IHI, was to reduce Caesarian section rates by 30 percent or more within a year. The experts brought best practices to the effort, including an assumption from the start that each patient would seek to have a vaginal birth rather than defaulting—as some patients were doing—to a Caesarian. Increased nursing support as well as the ready availability of anesthesia also helped lift the incidence of vaginal births. The timing of certain procedures proved crucial. Two specific procedures that elevate the likelihood of a C-section are electively inducing labor before the patient is at term (before thirty-seven weeks) and administering spinal anesthesia early in labor. By reducing these practices when not medically necessary, the incidence of C-sections declines.

The results were encouraging: within twelve months, 15 percent of the organizations reduced their Caesarian section rates by 25 percent or more, and 50 percent of the organizations achieved reductions of from 10 to 25 percent.

> It was clear we were really on to something [says Berwick]. I think maybe one third of the hospitals actually made a reduction in Caesarian sections; today we'd regard that as a not very successful effort, but we definitely were getting new ideas out. . . . Early results were that about one out of every three teams made very substantial progress. As we got better at it, by the fifth or sixth or seventh *Breakthrough Series,* we were up to two out of three teams making substantial progress.

In a similar Breakthrough Series effort concerning congestive heart failure, significant improvements were achieved by managing patients' conditions closely at home. Patients were taught to self-manage by getting on a scale daily and reporting weight gains right away to a nurse—who would make rapid adjustments in medications based on the change. Through careful management, at-home patients avoid the slide into a worsening condition and thus stay out of the hospital.

Hospitals sent small teams to three two-day sessions in which participants learned not only from leading experts but also from one another. The participants would take what they gained at the learning sessions back to their hospitals to test various ideas in a clinical setting. Some months later, they would return and report results. "The key was to combine subject matter experts in specific clinical areas with application experts who could help organizations select, test, and implement changes on the front lines of care," says Maureen Bisognano. There were *Breakthrough* projects on Caesarian section rates, neonatal intensive care, cardiac surgery, asthma care, low-back pain, adverse drug events, and many more. There was no limit to the clinical subjects clinicians could learn about from experts or one another. "We could yell out to the country, 'Let's work on asthma, let's work on heart surgery' . . . and we'd have twenty, forty, a hundred organizations sign up," says Berwick.

These were real, tangible achievements; achievements that, slowly but surely, demonstrated that this new organization might well have staying power; might well play a role in the movement to transform the quality of care in America.

3

The Annenberg
Conference on Error

———◦◦◦◦———

"What would it take for hospitals
to become high-reliability organizations?"

Lucian Leape, MD, is tall and thin, a distinguished-looking gentle-
man in his seventies, with a warm, approachable manner. He is
widely recognized as one of the leading experts in the country—the
world, really—on error in medicine. As he sits in his unpretentious
office at the Harvard School of Public Health in Boston, he recalls
with evident fondness his days a half century earlier in the medical
school a block away.

"I loved medical school," says Leape, beaming at the memory of his
days at Harvard in the 1950s. "I absolutely loved every day." Leape
trained in surgery at Massachusetts General and Children's Hospital
in Boston, earning board certification in three surgical specialties:

general, thoracic, and pediatric. He was in a hurry not only to put his skills to work but to do so in an environment where the clinical demands were nonstop. He searched for the busiest pediatric hospitals he could find and settled upon Alder Hey in Liverpool, England, then the largest pediatric hospital in Europe.

"There were life-threatening conditions almost every day," he recalls. "There were a lot of patients with severe congenital malformations of the esophagus, lungs, intestines, urinary tract." These difficult problems afflicting babies required great surgical skill. Day after day, Leape remained in the operating room fixing one baby after another. "It was a grueling schedule, but we were really saving lives," he says. "The parents would be so grateful—it was wonderful."

Leape eventually found his way back to Boston working at New England Medical Center and teaching at Tufts Medical School. He practiced and taught successfully for many years, but by the mid-1980s, he had grown weary of what seemed endless turf battles within academic medicine. Since he was also suffering from burnout, he thought of making a change—a *significant* change. He was drawn to health policy, and seeing that it was dominated by economists, Leape thought that as a doctor he might be able to contribute something. And so it was that, at age fifty-five, Lucian Leape packed up and moved to California to spend the academic year at the RAND Corporation mid-career program in health policy. There was something anomalous about this. Leape had always been comfortable disseminating knowledge and now he was a student himself; indeed, his classmates, graduate students from UCLA, were in the same age group as his own children. Leape studied economics, statistics, health policy, and health education.

"At RAND I got an appreciation for what the issues in health policy were, and I got the grounding in basic evaluative sciences that I needed," Leape says. "I didn't become a statistician, but I learned enough to talk with a statistician intelligently. I learned a fair amount about health services research, techniques which I had known nothing about." His mentor was the head of the program, Robert Brook, MD, who also oversees the Robert Wood Johnson Foundation Clinical Scholars Program at RAND. After completing the RAND program, Leape returned to Boston and began work on a monograph concerning unnecessary surgery.

Back in Boston, Leape and Berwick met for the first time and Berwick came away impressed with Leape's eloquence, intellect, and energy. During this time, Leape also met Berwick's close friend Howard Hiatt, MD, former dean of the Harvard School of Public Health, who had initiated a study in New York State to gain a deeper understanding of error in medicine. It would be the largest study of its kind, and Hiatt invited Leape to join the team. To start with, Leape worked with colleagues to define essential terms such as adverse event—"an injury caused, at least in part, by medical management (including failure to manage or diagnose), which produced measurable disability (at least an additional day in the hospital) and was unintended." They defined negligence as "failure to meet standards reasonably expected of the average physician."

After about a year of preparatory work, the research team was ready to go into the field. Leape would travel across New York State running training sessions for local doctors who would actually conduct the work of reviewing records. During most of 1989, Leape and colleagues studied the records of more than 30,000 randomly selected patients who had been discharged in 1984 from fifty-one randomly selected hospitals throughout the state.

After processing and reviewing the data, Leape was shocked by the results. The study found that "nearly 4 percent of patients suffered an injury that prolonged their hospital stay or resulted in measurable disability" and that nearly 14 percent of those injuries were fatal. The study found that 69 percent of the injuries were due to errors that Leape saw as clearly preventable. The implications were frightening: Projecting from the results Leape estimated that every year in the United States 120,000 people were dying from *preventable* medical errors.

"When I saw the data that two-thirds of the injuries were due to mistakes I was stunned!" exclaims Leape. He and Troy Brennan, a physician at Brigham and Women's, wrote up the results for two articles published in the *New England Journal of Medicine (NEJM)* in January 1991.

Leape awaited the fury from the medical world, the shock and determination to do whatever was necessary to solve the problem. A front page story in the *New York Times* affirmed the significant news value of the work. And then . . . *nothing.* "Absolutely no reaction," Leape recalls. "It died."

How could that be? How could the largest study of its kind by highly qualified physicians and sponsored by such a prestigious institution generate such shocking findings that were essentially ignored by the medical community throughout the country? In a way, the nature of the results prevented the study from having the kind of impact it should have. The numbers were so large and disturbing that many people in health care simply didn't believe it. It was, after all, only one study, and one that directly contradicted the bedrock belief that American health care was of the highest possible quality— surely the finest in the world. This was not so much a suspicion or belief as it was an article of faith. It would take more than one study, no matter how compelling, to shift perception concerning the safety and quality of American health care. Perhaps as much as anything it was, as Leape defines it, the widely held belief that it's *just the way it is,* that when you perform difficult or complicated procedures sometimes things go wrong. In fact, says Leape, "most doctors who reacted indicated they thought our results were pretty good!"

Leape was more energized than disappointed, though, for he had discovered his new calling: researching and studying medical error.

He delved into a pilot study at Mass General and the Brigham to identify system failures—as opposed to individual mistakes—behind medication errors (the study was conducted in 1992 with David Bates, another physician at Brigham and Women's Hospital). Leape would find that medication errors accounted for the largest group of errors in medicine—a significant discovery.

While the study was underway, Leape worked on a paper he called "Error in Medicine." He had begun it in 1990 when the Harvard Medical Practice Study was still being analyzed, and he had continued working on it for more than a year. As part of his research on the paper, Leape went to the Harvard Medical Library and searched for material on error prevention in health care. He found nothing. With the assistance of a librarian, he broadened the error prevention search to engineering and humanities databases—and dozens of references popped up. He had discovered "a whole new world outside health care," the world of industrial quality control that Batalden and Berwick had earlier discovered, and with that discovery, Lucian Leape's view of health care changed forever.

"I discovered a whole world of people thinking analytically about how you prevent mistakes," he recalls. "There are a lot of applications in aviation, for example. They'd done a fantastic job and it seemed to me that there were similarities between doctors and pilots—both think they're pretty special people—and I got really excited. It seemed really relevant and I thought, 'This is what I'm looking for.'"

"Error in Medicine" was published in the *Journal of the American Medical Association* (*JAMA*) on the day before Christmas, 1994. The article received little attention upon publication, but it was not long before it would gain recognition as one of the most important pieces of writing in the new quality movement. Leape made it clear that he had become an apostle of continuous quality as preached by Deming and practiced by industry. Leape wrote that in "the culture of medical

practice . . . there is a powerful emphasis on perfection, both in diagnosis and treatment." Further, he wrote,

> Role models in medical education reinforce the concept of infallibil-
> ity. . . . Errors are rarely admitted or discussed among physicians in
> private practice. Physicians typically feel, not without reason, that ad-
> mission of error will lead to censure or increased surveillance or,
> worse, that their colleagues will regard them as incompetent or care-
> less. Far better to conceal a mistake or, if that's impossible, to try to
> shift blame to another, even the patient.

And yet, Leape wrote, the notion that perfection was somehow
achievable for doctors was nonsensical. All clinicians were human and
knew that mistakes were inevitable. The influence of industrial quality
techniques on Leape's thinking was evident. "While the proximal error
leading to an accident is, in fact, usually a 'human error,' the causes of
that error are often well beyond the individual's control," he wrote. "All
humans err frequently. Systems that rely on error-free performance are
doomed to fail. . . . The primary objective of system design for safety is
to *make it difficult for individuals to err* [emphasis added]." Leape
noted that in the airline industry, for example, engineers "assume that
errors and failures are inevitable and design systems to 'absorb' them."

The power of Leape's essay lay in the force of its simple argument:
*Error prevention systems work brilliantly in various industries. If we
adapt these systems in healthcare, we will reduce error, improve quality,
and save lives.* No one could argue with Leape's contention that
"physicians should not have to rely on their memories to retrieve a
laboratory test result, and nurses should not have to remember the
time a medication dose is due . . . tasks that computers do much
more reliably than humans."

In 1995, Leape and his colleague David Bates delved deeply into the
issue of medication errors in a study at Mass General and the Brigham.

They found that the rate of adverse drug events at those hospitals was *ten times* higher than reported. The research demonstrated that the majority of adverse drug events result from system failures. The timing of this paper, published just months after "Error in Medicine" and a series of serious errors in early 1995, only added to Leape's growing stature as a leading expert on error in medicine.

Barely more than a month after Leape's "Error in Medicine" paper was published, the Dana-Farber Cancer Institute announced the discovery of the medication error that had killed Betsy Lehman. Suddenly, Leape's *JAMA* essay seemed prescient. The timing that had seemed so off weeks earlier was now fortuitous. Throughout the medical world, clinicians, administrators, and academics were asking the same troubling question: How could such a terrible mistake have been made at Dana-Farber?

In the months after the revelation about the Betsy Lehman overdose, leading officials in American medicine engaged in intense discussions about how to respond. One of those officials was Martin Hatlie, MD, of the American Medical Association (AMA) who oversaw the AMA program on how to mitigate malpractice. Another major official in American medicine thinking about how to respond constructively was Dennis O'Leary, MD, chairman of the Joint Commission. That spring, the AMA and Joint Commission got together with the American Association for the Advancement of Science and the Annenberg Center and agreed to host a conference on error in medicine. The historic meeting in October, 1996, at the Annenberg Center for Health Sciences in Rancho Mirage, California, was titled "Examining Errors in Health Care: Developing a Prevention, Education and Research Agenda."

Lucian Leape had been largely ignored when he and Troy Brennan and colleagues had produced the Harvard Medical Practice Study, but he wasn't being ignored anymore: He was selected to give the keynote address at the Annenberg Conference while Don Berwick was chosen to deliver the plenary address.

The timing of the conference was ideal. Drawn to Rancho Mirage for the event were doctors, nurses, technicians, academics, and medical administrators, in addition to experts from various other industries—all concerned with safety in health care. The opening sentence in the conference program stated that "despite remarkable advances in almost every field of medicine, an age-old problem continues to haunt medical care—the occurrence of errors." At the time, this was revolutionary stuff. Never before had such prestigious mainstream organizations gathered for the specific purpose of acknowledging and dealing with the widespread existence of errors in medicine.

In addition to Leape, Berwick, and others, one of the conference speakers was James Reason, professor of psychology at the University of Manchester in England, and the author of the well-regarded book *Human Error*, published in 1990. Reason got the attention of the audience when he said that it was "natural for us to believe that disastrous accidents must be due to equally monstrous blunders. But the close investigation of organizational accidents has a way of turning conventional wisdom on its head. . . . The best people can make the worst mistakes. The greatest calamities can happen to conscientious and well-run organizations." It was about systems, Reason argued, not individuals.

The most emotional moment at the conference came when the story of a seven-year-old named Ben Kolb was told. Ben had gone into Martin Memorial Hospital in Stuart, Florida, for routine ear surgery; after being injected with the wrong drug, he died. The reaction to this tragic event by the hospital and doctors was highly unusual: They came forward, told the family exactly what had happened, hid nothing, and told the truth about the entire painful episode. At the Annenberg Conference the story was greeted with tears and thunderous applause, and although Leape was as moved by the story as anyone, he thought the audience response constituted a scathing indictment of the reality in health care. He thought that telling the truth about errors ought to be the norm.

When Leape rose to deliver the keynote address he was helping to break new ground in the quality movement. Until Leape's work with Brennan, Bates and others, the new quality movement had focused on process improvement toward better quality. With his laser-like focus on error, Leape added a new and urgently needed dimension to the movement. Through Leape's efforts, safety was recognized as a sine qua non of quality. In the years ahead, the concept of real quality would elude some health care stakeholders (particularly those who thought having "the best bone guy in town" defined quality). But *everyone* understood error.

It had taken Leape a few days to prepare his remarks, yet the insights and wisdom contained in his address were years in the making. It had been two years—nearly to the day—since Betsy Lehman had entered the Dana-Farber Cancer Institute, and Leape opened by dedicating his remarks to her. "In a real sense," he said, "our meeting here . . . is proof that she did not die in vain." Leape noted that Betsy's death was followed "by reports of other medical catastrophes: amputation of a wrong limb, breast, operation on wrong side of the head. The public began to ask, 'What is wrong?'"

The numbers were sobering, he noted. Extrapolating from the Harvard Medical Practice Study, Leape estimated that there were 1 million preventable medical errors in the United States each year, resulting in more than 100,000 deaths. The cost of these injuries Leape estimated at $33 billion annually. Why, then, had so very little been done in health care to address the error problem? The disturbing answer was ignorance: a lack of awareness. *No one measured, so no one knew.* "Until recent reports, most hospitals and doctors did not honestly believe that error was much of a problem in health care," said Leape. "Even now, after a series of reported catastrophes, most hospitals have no idea of the extent of their error problem."

Part of the reason was that no one measured and studied, but another important reason was that most error data was self-reported and Leape had found that self-reporting invariably results in drastic undercounting of errors. When error reports were done independently—by observation or review of records—the reported rate of errors was from twenty to thirty times self-reported rates.

Leape noted that many hospitals and physicians were pleased with a 90 percent success rate with certain procedures. "But 90 percent success is a 10 percent defect rate—a level that *no* industry would tolerate." He cited a study conducted in five states to determine how frequently Medicare diabetes patients received the testing needed to manage the disease. Only 16 percent received a hemoglobin A1c test, 46 percent got a retinal exam, and 55 percent received a test of serum cholesterol. Leape observed that defect rates this high—from 45 to 84 percent—were scandalous; indeed, they would be considered absurd by industries for which defect rates of 1 percent were considered unacceptable.

As the quality movement gained traction during the 1990s, there came a common refrain: Health care is different from other industries because every patient is different, but Leape rebuts that: "It's not *patient* variations we're talking about. It's *our* variations that are the problem—defects in *our* performance."

Like Batalden and Berwick, Leape believed that the medical culture, which discouraged the disclosure of errors, actually worked against overall quality improvement. Transparency enables the medical community to learn from mistakes and improve care. Concealing mistakes slows the improvement process and ill serves patients. "I believe our judgmental approach to error—blaming and punishing—is the major barrier to effective error reduction in our health-care institutions, because it keeps us from knowing when they occur and why they occur," Leape told the audience. The body of scientific work produced by cognitive psychologists and human factors experts was powerfully instructive for health care, he said, in that the experts identified simple truths about error—that even the most competent people frequently make mistakes and that errors often occur as a result of interruptions and distractions. To many in the audience, this was a way of thinking they had never before even considered. But Leape informed them that pioneers in the quality movement had been thinking this way for many years.

He wondered about establishing an environment in which clinicians were free to disclose errors so that the larger community could learn from them, thus improving patient care. He asked pointedly: "What needs to be done to make error prevention a top priority objective? . . . What would it take for hospitals to become high-reliability organizations?"

Leape's admonition to "look beyond the individual to the systems they work in" was being taken quite seriously in some quarters. Coincidentally with the Annenberg Conference, the *New England Journal of Medicine* ran a series of articles on quality of care. The very existence of the series in the *NEJM* was not only unusual but also a powerful signal to the medical world that the new quality movement had broken through to mainstream medicine. In the first installment of the series, published just a few weeks before the Annenberg conference, David Blumenthal, MD, of Massachusetts General Hospital, wrote that different stakeholders within health care had quite different perspectives on what constituted quality. Although "physicians tend to see quality in terms of the excellence of the services they provide ('doing the right things right') and the quality of their interactions with patients," employees, insurers and others define quality differently. Doctors tended to see quality through the lens of an individual encounter with a patient, but others saw quality resulting from "the optimal functioning of systems."

Blumenthal thought that few physicians were ready for the move toward systemization. Although many clinicians dismissed the notion that quality in health care was measurable, the *NEJM* was using its clout to send an unequivocal message: Reliable scientific methods had been developed to measure the quality of care. In part 2 of the series, Robert H. Brook, MD, and Elizabeth A. McGlynn, PhD, both of RAND, and Paul D. Cleary, a Harvard Medical School PhD, made an emphatic statement:

> We now have sophisticated and efficient methods of measuring quality that can help clinicians and institutions improve the quality of the medical care they provide. . . . Tools are now available to measure quality efficiently. Our goal should be to ensure that all patients receive care considered to be high in quality on the basis of scientific data and expert judgment.

The twin events—the *NEJM* series along with the Annenberg Conference and its support from the very mainstream AMA—were signs of slow but certain progress. And the pace of that progress would soon accelerate.

4

To Err Is Human

"Before this I was concerned.
Now I am radicalized."

In the middle and late 1990s, the spread of managed care through-out the country triggered a political backlash as the news media car-ried countless stories about insurance companies coldly denying patients critical care. Physicians complained bitterly that insurers had seized control of the health care system, deciding, often in an ir-rational manner, who would receive treatment and who would not. Citing a chorus of complaints from doctors and patients, the press portrayed insurers as having a choke hold on the American health care system. Managed care—invented to try and bring some level of sanity to spiraling costs—had become the villain.

In an attempt to address patient concerns, state and federal elected officials, along with physician groups and consumer advocates, proposed enactment of a national patients' bill of rights. In March 1997, the Clinton administration appointed a Presidential Commission to study managed care and quality. Co-chaired by Donna Shalala, secretary of health and human services, and Alexis Herman, secretary of labor, the President's Advisory Commission on Consumer Protection and Quality in the Health Care Industry was charged with writing a patients' bill of rights that would draw a clear protective line for consumers against managed care.

As the commission was being formed, Don and Ann Berwick, along with their two youngest children, were spending a sabbatical year in Alaska while Ann worked as an environmental lawyer in the state attorney general's office. Don Berwick—via phone, computer, and regular return trips to Cambridge—continued running IHI from Anchorage.

While in Alaska, Berwick received an unexpected phone call from the White House. The caller explained that the president was appointing a commission to explore a variety of aspects of healthcare, including quality, and asked whether Berwick would be interested in participating. Berwick accepted, thrilled to be asked. The invitation was an affirmation that Berwick and IHI had made important strides in the new quality movement. Beyond that, it was an opportunity for Berwick to bring all that he had learned to a committee with real clout. He began to travel regularly from Anchorage to Washington and soon became fully engaged in the project.

After some time, the commission decided to produce an interim report—*Consumer Bill of Rights and Responsibilities*—which it released in November 1997. Commission members gathered in Washington as President Clinton spoke about how significant the bill of rights would be to consumers. The new document sought to assure consumers the right to "accurate, easily understood information," a choice of health care providers, a voice in treatment decisions, confidentiality, and more. On the surface, it appeared the commission had done its job—protect patients from predatory managed care practices.

Under the surface, however, the story was quite different. Though it was an article of faith at the time that managed care was the problem, there was mounting evidence that the larger issue in health care was quality. "RAND was showing that problems of quality were rampant—basically universal," says Berwick. Though the political sizzle was about the bill of rights, the commission's charge to report on the general state of quality in American health care was of greater consequence.

After delivering the bill of rights interim document, the committee significantly broadened the scope of its work to encompass quality care in general. This, of course, excited Berwick, and the opportunity to make a real impact also motivated other committee members. There was a diligence about the committee and their devotion to the work that impressed Berwick. The group met about a dozen times, and for every session at least one, and usually both, of the cabinet members were in attendance.

Essential to the committee's work was gathering the best data on the level of quality care in the United States, and that came from the scholars at RAND. A key moment came when Elizabeth A. McGlynn, PhD, director of the Center for Research on Quality in Health Care at RAND, testified before the commission. McGlynn—along with her RAND colleagues, among them Mark Schuster and Robert Brook—was conducting an ongoing study of quality, and her conclusions were grim. She told the commission that in the United States "there are no guarantees about the quality of care any individual is likely to receive for any particular medical problem."

This was a jarring assertion and clearly contrary to the widely held assumption that health care quality in the United States was generally superb and surely the finest in the world. But that was not at all the case, McGlynn testified. She identified three distinct types of quality issues: overuse, underuse, and errors. "Overuse occurs when a patient is given an intervention for which the expected risks substantially exceed the expected benefits," she told the commission. "Underuse is the failure to provide services when the expected benefits are greater than the expected risks. Errors are mistakes in the provision of services that have the potential to result in serious adverse consequences for the patient."

As commission members listened attentively, McGlynn listed numerous examples of each, starting with overuse. She cited a study among a Medicare population revealing that 14 percent of coronary artery bypass graft surgeries were deemed inappropriate, and an additional 30 percent were "of uncertain clinical value." Often, she said, children suffering frequent ear infections received tympanostomy tubes to improve drainage. A study McGlynn cited "found that 23 percent of requests to insert tympanostomy tubes were clinically inappropriate and an additional 36 percent were of questionable clinical utility." She said there existed an epidemic of antibiotic misuse for viral infections where it is known that such treatment has zero impact and yet, in some cases, as many as 70 percent of patients received antibiotics for a viral infection.

McGlynn cited widespread underuse of preventive care, including data indicating that about one third of children in more than 300 managed care plans did *not* receive recommended immunizations by the age of two—truly fundamental elements of quality care. Although 95 percent of children received the proper immunizations in some plans, there were also plans in which only 20 percent received them. McGlynn told of a similar story with screenings for breast, cervical, and colon cancer.

Among the most troubling forms of underuse involved chronic diseases. McGlynn noted that essential treatments for diabetics included a dilated eye examination, yet "an average of 38 percent of persons with diabetes enrolled in the 330 managed care plans reporting to the National Committee for Quality Assurance (NCQA) had an eye examination in the past year with a range from 10 percent to 75 percent among individual plans." Like so much of the data Mc-Glynn presented to the commission, this was a stunning statistic. It meant that an average of 62 percent of diabetics were *not* receiving a critically important eye examination. It meant there were plans in which 90 percent of participants were not receiving the exam. This was a level of neglect difficult to imagine in a modern health care system. McGlynn found that patients who received life-saving beta blockers "had a 43 percent lower rate of mortality than those who did not"; but in a New Jersey study of Medicare patients, 79 percent did *not* receive beta blockers within ninety days of a heart attack.

She found widespread and inexplicable variations in the quality of care. "The evidence from the variations literature," she said, referring to work pioneered by Jack Wennberg, MD, and his colleagues at Dartmouth, "is the 'smoking gun' that underscores the likelihood of wide disparities in the quality of care." Surgical procedures in various parts of the country showed wide variation; in one study among an affluent population at one community hospital, the Caesarian section rates ranged from 19 percent to 42 percent, depending upon the obstetrician.

One problem affecting quality care, McGlynn observed, was the often slow spread of new and useful knowledge to clinicians. She noted that publications with practice guidelines—channels for conveying new information to doctors about best practices—had gone from just one a year between 1975 and 1980 to 454 a year between 1993 and 1997. Her conclusion was emphatic: "There is a gap between best practices and actual practices." There was something particularly unsettling about this conclusion. Wasn't it true that American doctors relied on scientific evidence—the most *advanced* scientific evidence—for their chosen treatments? If a certain treatment was known to be the best—had been proven scientifically to be the best—how could it not be applied to every patient? How was it possible that so many patients received treatments different from or less than what was known to be the best treatment? McGlynn noted that industrial quality techniques could help increase the use of best practices.

Berwick was deeply impressed with the work of McGlynn and her RAND colleagues, and he was pleased to hear her talk of system improvement and quality techniques from other industries. This, after all, was precisely what he and IHI were working on. In mid-March, 1998, the commission delivered its report, *Quality First: Better Healthcare for All Americans,* to President Clinton. It had none of the sex appeal of the patients' bill of rights the commission had delivered four months earlier, but it contained far more substance.

"That report was a very important turning point for lots of us," recalls Berwick, "because, although Clinton had started this thinking that the problem was managed care—that managed care was out of control with these vicious organizations that would hurt anyone to make money—that wasn't what we concluded. The commission concluded we have a really serious systemic problem. I think that changed a lot of minds."

The commission's quality of care indictment found that "while most Americans receive high-quality care, too many patients receive substandard care. Quality problems include wide variation in health care services, underuse of some services and overuse of others, and an unacceptable level of errors . . . [that] too many Americans are injured during the course of their treatment, and some die prematurely as a result"; that millions more "do not receive necessary care and suffer needless complications that add to health care costs and reduce productivity." The report stated bluntly that health care stakeholders "must make quality improvement the driving force of the industry."

It was a clear and much needed call to action, certainly hospital administrators, clinicians, and others—all with patients' well-being uppermost in mind—would grasp the report and charge forward toward reform. In fact, to Berwick's surprise, very few did so. How, he wondered, could such an indictment, backed by so much data, be shunted aside? It was a moment when Berwick and others could have seen the lack of reaction to a presidential commission and walked away, gone off in other directions seeking work that might have more of an impact.

Of course, they did nothing of the sort. Instead, they moved forward, convinced that focusing on quality would yield huge dividends. And very quickly, immediately after the president's commission was disbanded, they were given a new platform on which to conduct their work. For the leadership of the Institute of Medicine of the National Academies also recognized the unfinished business on quality. The institute launched the Quality of Health Care in America project in June 1998 "with the charge of developing a strategy that will result in a *threshold improvement* in quality over the next ten years." The idea was to produce a series of reports that would pave the way for significant quality improvement in American health care. The members of the Committee were a distinguished group chaired by William C. Richardson, president and CEO of the W. K. Kellogg Foundation. This group of distinguished and accomplished people, with Berwick and Leape playing central roles, would soon produce two of the most important documents in the history of American health care.

But before they did so, it became amply clear that the events of 1998 marked it as a crucial period in the new quality movement. The presidential commission's scathing report on the quality of care was released in March. Just a few months later, Beth McGlynn's RAND study findings appeared as an article in the *Milbank Quarterly*, soon followed by *JAMA*'s publication of "The Report of the Roundtable on Quality," a document produced by an Institute of Medicine (IOM) National Roundtable on Health Care Quality led by Mark R. Chassin, MD, and Robert W. Galvin, the chairman of Motorola. Chassin was the former New York State Health Commissioner, and Galvin had a national reputation in the industrial quality movement. The report carried a succinct—and striking—conclusion: "The quality of health care can be precisely defined and measured with a degree of scientific accuracy comparable with that of most measures used in clinical medicine. Serious and widespread quality problems exist throughout American medicine."

Though the Roundtable report and the presidential commission received little public attention, "they did lead to greater professional awareness," says Berwick. "The Roundtable report was very important. David Lawrence, CEO of Kaiser Permanente at the time, had enormous credibility, and when he said that the problem with American health care was not small—'the chassis is broken'—that got people in the industry to sit up and take notice."

This was among the most productive periods ever in the new quality movement—a six-month period in 1998 during which two gold-plated groups of quality experts issued the most sweeping indictment of the health care system in modern times.

Just as 1998 had been a historic year for the new quality movement, so too would 1999 be a landmark year, but for very private reasons, within the Berwick family. Don Berwick had devoted his professional life to the pursuit of quality in health care. By 1999, Berwick had seen the health care system from every conceivable angle, it seemed, but now he was about to have a very different view of the system—one that would inform his point of view as never before.

Ann Berwick was fifty-one years old in the spring of 1999, had enjoyed a successful career as an attorney, and had recently competed in a twenty-eight-kilometer cross-country ski race in Alaska. Soon thereafter, however, something terrible happened: Ann developed symptoms of a rare autoimmune spinal cord problem. Two months after the ski race, Ann Berwick, as her husband recalled, "couldn't walk across our bedroom." Thus began an urgent—often chaotic and nearly always frustrating—journey through the catacombs of the American health care system. Initially, Don Berwick was reluctant to discuss it publicly, but he soon realized that the experience "resonates so thoroughly with the mission of improving health care that not to learn from it . . . seems wrong." With Ann's permission, he told the story in a December 1999 speech to the Eleventh Annual IHI National Forum on Quality Improvement in Health Care. The experience confirmed for Berwick what he knew to be true from his own years as a physician—that the people who work in health care, from doctors and nurses to technicians and pharmacists, bring an overriding sense of "goodwill, kindness, generosity, commitment, and dignity" to their work. But there was another side of the story. "Every hour of our care reminded me, and alerted Ann, about the enormous, costly, and painful gaps between what we got in our days of need and what we needed."

"From April through September Ann had six hospitalizations for a total of more than sixty inpatient days in three institutions, while she gradually experienced increasing pain, lost the ability to walk, and became essentially bedridden," Berwick recalls. He mentions his friend Lucian Leape's breakthrough research on medication errors:

Now I have seen [errors] firsthand . . . sitting by Ann's bedside for week after week of acute care. The errors were not rare; they were the norm. During one admission, the neurologist told us in the morning, "By no means should you be getting anticholinergic agents," and a medication with profound anticholinergic side effects was given that afternoon. The attending neurologist in another admission told us by phone that a crucial and potentially toxic drug should be started immediately. He said, "Time is of the essence." That was on Thursday morning at 10:00 A.M. The first dose was given sixty hours later—on

Saturday night at 10:00 P.M. Nothing I could do, nothing I did, nothing I could think of made any difference. It nearly drove me mad. Colace was discontinued by a physician's order on day one, and was nonetheless brought by the nurse every single evening throughout a fourteen-day admission. Ann was supposed to receive five intravenous doses of a very toxic chemotherapy agent, but dose three was labeled as dose two. For half a day, no record could be found that dose two had ever been given, even though I had watched it drip in myself. I will tell you from my personal observation: no day passed—not one—without a medication error. Most weren't serious, but they scared us.

We needed consistent, reliable information, based, we would have hoped, on the best science available. Instead we often heard a cacophony of meaningless and sometimes contradictory conclusions. Ann received Cytoxan [the drug, in massive overdose, that had killed Betsy Lehman], which causes hair loss and low white blood cell count. *When would these occur?* We asked. The answers varied by a factor of five. Drugs tried and proven futile in one admission would be recommended in the next as if they were fresh ideas. . . . During one crucial phase of diagnosis, one doctor told us to hope that the diagnosis would be of a certain disease, because that disease has a benign course. That same evening, another doctor told us to hope for the opposite, because that same disease is relentless—sometimes fatal.

In one case, Ann's sleeping medication was administered at 8:00 P.M., even though she was going to bed two hours later. In another instance, sleeping medications were administered at 3:00 A.M. and she was then awakened at 4:00 A.M. to have her blood pressure checked. Transitions were particularly jarring. A physician new to Ann's case asked how long she had been suffering from MS—though she did not have MS.

Fortunately, after many months, Ann began to recover, but the experience had been traumatic. "Before this I was concerned," says Berwick. "Now I am radicalized. If what happened to Ann could happen in our best institutions, I wonder more than ever before what the average must be like."

The timing of Ann's illness coincided with her husband's beginning work on a new IOM committee that would soon make history. When the committee convened in the spring of 1998 it was not clear initially what aspect of quality the group would take on. Committee members discussed the possibility of doing another general report on quality, but recognized there was no point. They had just done that with the President's Advisory Commission Report, which echoed both the Roundtable report published in *JAMA* and McGlynn's RAND work. Berwick's frustration grew out of the reality that not enough attention, within the medical community or outside it, had been paid to any of this work. The status quo reigned and as long as that was true change would be all but impossible. And then came one of those somewhat magical moments when an idea was formed—a perfect idea at the right moment. Rather than putting out yet another report on the unfortunate state of quality generally, the idea was to focus a report specifically on errors—on mistakes that harmed patients. In large measure, the work had been done for them. The Harvard Medical Practice Study by Leape and his colleagues was a landmark document, yet it had received little attention since its publication nearly a decade earlier. And, more recently, a study in Utah and Colorado had reached similar conclusions.

During the committee's deliberations, members grappled with the issue of how to gain attention for their cause. The issue, Berwick thought, was not that there was insufficient evidence to suggest the country had a serious problem with medical errors. The jury was long since in on that question. The more difficult issue was how the committee could persuade people to pay attention so that they could begin to solve the problem. At one point, the committee invited a group of journalists to meet for a day-long session with the hope that committee members might gain a better understanding of how the media worked and how the committee could attract coverage for its cause. Committee members met with more than a dozen reporters and editors from a variety of news organizations, including PBS, NBC, the *Washington Post,* the *New York Times,* the *Wall Street Journal,* and the *Boston Globe.* The journalists told the committee that they should learn from the managed care story and focus on a villain and a victim. That, however, was precisely what the committee members wanted to avoid. "The last thing you want to do with safety is say this is the fault of the providers," says Janet Corrigan, the committee staff director. "We were trying to make crystal clear that the *system* was the problem."

Dubbed *To Err Is Human: Building a Safer Health System,* the report took shape as the committee worked for about a year. Toward the end, committee members—and Berwick and Leape were in the thick of this—worked closely with staff, going through eight or ten drafts of the executive summary to get it just right. The report stated bluntly that "the goal of this report is to break [the] cycle of inaction. The status quo is not acceptable and cannot be tolerated any longer . . . it is simply not acceptable for patients to be harmed by the same health care system that is supposed to offer healing and comfort."

The report was quite open in stating that the committee aspired to influence the public to put pressure on the system—on doctors, health plans, administrators—on everyone involved with maintaining the status quo. It was clear the committee was frustrated that work by Leape and others had not triggered the appropriate outrage. By highlighting the error problem, the committee believed they could win over the public; in effect, they hoped that patients throughout the country not only would stand up and take notice as never before but would develop an intolerance for errors so pronounced that it would force hospitals to institute safer practices. The committee pointedly noted that there were essentially no external pressures in health care at the time, no sense of outrage or intolerance by the public at all. Thus, hospitals did not feel compelled to change.

The report quickly got to what the commissioners considered the heart of the matter: that the problem of safety was not about individual clinicians but about whole systems. The report noted that "health care is a decade or more behind other high-risk industries in its attention to ensuring basic safety." This was a puzzling anomaly. How could so many of the country's brightest people work within a system that was so fundamentally unsound? With so many smart people in health care, and with so much advanced technology used in medical procedures, it was not only ironic but utterly counterintuitive that health care was decades behind other industries in the use of modern information technology and techniques for quality control. This was the core problem—as well as the most tantalizing opportunity.

But the opportunity could be realized only if people paid attention to the report, and that required some sort of news hook to capture the imagination of the press and public. Janet Corrigan, an accomplished PhD with an impressive professional background, came up with the answer. One evening, as she was working on the Executive Summary, trying to find a way to define the magnitude of the problem, she started playing with the numbers. She took the two defining error studies—the Utah/Colorado study and the Leape Harvard Medical Practice Study—and began to scribble some extrapolations based on the data. The question in her mind was this: If the deaths in those studies due to errors were applied to the United States as a whole, what would the result look like? After some quick math, she had her answer. Extrapolating from the two studies, she concluded that each year in the United States between 44,000 and 98,000 Americans were killed by medical errors. (The higher number was close to Leape's widely ignored projection years earlier.) She looked up leading causes of death in the United States—motor vehicle accidents, cancer, and so forth—and found that fatal medical errors at the levels she had computed would rank about fifth. This left Corrigan all but speechless: "The idea that the health care system we create to help people—to cure and save them—was actually in and of itself a leading cause of death . . . "

After an exceptionally vigorous review process at the National Academies, more rigorous than usual given the explosive nature of the numbers, the report was approved for publication. When a news organization threatened to publish the report early, before others had a chance to receive it, the commission staff decided to accelerate the release.

"I remember getting woken up on a Sunday night [Thanksgiving weekend, 1999], I was scheduled to go in three days to Washington to release the report," recalls Berwick. "It was Janet [Corrigan] on the phone. She said, 'The report had been leaked. . . . They're not going to honor the embargo. We're going live tomorrow. Can you get down here?' So, I went down early Monday morning, Lucian and I on the same plane. That day was amazing." When Berwick and Leape arrived at National Airport, they were picked up and whisked to different network studios for interviews, and for the next three days the report dominated the news across the United States. Berwick, Leape, and Bill Richardson, the committee chair, were featured on every network and every major newspaper in the country.

"It was three days of saturation coverage," recalls Corrigan. So great was the interest that the National Academies Web site crashed under the hits. Berwick and Leape dazzled the media.

"They made it come alive with details," she says. "They became the two major public voices on the report." Says Leape: "The 98,000 number just blew people away."

Beneath the numbers of deaths, the report was rich with unsettling conclusions about the quality of care in the United States. The *Washington Post* front page article led with the 98,000 possible deaths, as did most publications. The *Wall Street Journal,* which also led with the 44,000 to 98,000 numbers, included a particularly potent and well crafted paragraph by reporter Ron Winslow:

> The report paints a disturbing picture of medical care in America in which patients are vulnerable not only to their illnesses but to a flawed health-care delivery system that is characterized by problems as mundane as sloppy handwriting on prescriptions and as complex as a torrent of new medical knowledge that leaves doctors and other practitioners struggling to keep up.

Interestingly, the spokesman for the American Hospital Association, Richard Wade, did not dispute the problem. Wade said: "What this report acknowledges is a need for better safeguards and systems for doctors and nurses and others to minimize the possibility of errors. Is the system we have now adequate? No, it is not."

Although the core message of the report—that safety is not about individuals but systems—was not mentioned in every article, it did receive prominent play in the major newspapers, including the *Post, Journal,* and *New York Times.* The news was so big that a number of papers were moved to editorialize about it. One of the most important articles published in the wake of the report appeared in the *Times* on December 5 with the headline: "Do No Harm; Breaking Down Medicine's Culture of Silence." Sheryl Gay Stolberg wrote with particular insight:

The culture of silence, and why it needs to be broken, was the unstated theme of a report that shook the medical profession last week. . . .

The idea that doctors make mistakes is, of course, nothing new. But the idea that mistakes can be prevented by changing systems has been slow to catch on, in part because doctors rarely talk openly about their errors. The pat explanation is that they are afraid of being disciplined, or sued. But it is not the whole truth, says Dr. Lucian Leape. . . .

"Physicians are taught that it's your job not to make a mistake," Dr. Leape said. "It's like a sin. The whole concept of error as sin, as a moral failing, is deeply ingrained in medicine, and it is very destructive. It means people cannot talk about it, because it is too painful."

Stolberg wrote that human error could be viewed as "negligence, a willful disregard for standards." Or it could be seen as a simple matter of "normal human frailty." In medicine the problem was much more the later than the former. Stolberg wrote that Berwick's view was that overwhelmingly medical mistakes were committed by, as Stolberg put it, "good doctors trying to do the right thing, working under conditions that do not account for the fact that they are human."

Berwick was thrilled with the success of *To Err Is Human,* in part because he believed it was important to get the message about errors out there, but also because he knew that its success could lead to a demand for designing a better system of care. That was the natural next step for the IOM—to take on the truly immense challenge of designing the architecture for a medical delivery system that was safer and produced a higher level of quality. The same committee that produced *To Err Is Human* would now tackle the question of redesigning the delivery system—a vast and complex undertaking. The idea was to produce a report so compelling that health care leaders throughout the country would eagerly adopt its philosophy and begin to implement it—with marvelous quality and safety results.

That report, *Crossing the Quality Chasm: A New Health System for the 21st Century,* serves as a kind of bible of the new quality movement. "There was tremendous pressure to get the *Chasm* report out," recalls Janet Corrigan. "Whereas *To Err* was aimed at the public and press, *Chasm* aimed at leadership in health care." Although Berwick was widely seen as central to the report, the group was a rare and outstanding team that included, among others, Leape, William C. Richardson, president and CEO of the W. K. Kellogg Foundation; Molly Joel Coye, MD, an information technology (IT) expert and senior vice president of the Lewin Group; Brent James, MD, from Intermountain; Lonnie R. Bristow, MD, former president of the AMA; and David Lawrence, MD, chairman and CEO of the Kaiser Foundation Health Plan. Advisors to the committee included George J. Isham, MD, of HealthPartners; James L. Reinertsen, MD, CareGroup; Thomas Nolan, PhD, an IHI process improvement consultant close to Berwick; as well as doctors Elliott Fisher and Jack Wennberg from Dartmouth. The committee was divided into two working subgroups with Berwick as chair of "Redesigning the Chassis"—after the term coined by David Lawrence of Kaiser (The other subgroup, "Creating an Environment for Quality in Health Care," was co-chaired by Molly Joel Coye and Chris Bisgard, MD).

The groups worked assiduously over many months, with Berwick cranking at an accelerated pace. He and his group at one point huddled at an Institute of Medicine retreat in Woods Hole on Cape Cod, isolated with peace, quiet, and enormous intellectual energy. The question before Berwick's subcommittee was what the new system should look like. This was an opportunity for which Berwick had been waiting for more than twenty years. It was his job to lead a small subcommittee toward a prescription for how to remake American health care to dramatically improve quality. Don Berwick had never been more ready for anything in his life. During the morning there was some discussion and then came one of those flashes of light, a moment when all the work and thinking and reading and studying suddenly come together and the answer is clear. Berwick got up and went to the flipchart.

"Here's what we need," he said, starting to write on the chart. "We need a system that produces care that is safe, effective, patient-centered, prompt, efficient and equitable." And then he turned to the group and said, "How about these as goals?" And someone said, "Not prompt, how about timely?"

"So we wrote these things up there. . . . We spent two days defining that and then saying how would you get there? Describe the system that will get us there," Berwick says. It would prove to be a moment of pure inspiration, for central to *Chasm* were precisely the goals enunciated that day by Berwick. The very wording that Berwick scrawled on that chart was the final language in the *Chasm* report. Since then it has been quoted in thousands of articles and books throughout the world as the standard to which health care should aspire. *Crossing the Quality Chasm* was among the most sweeping and ambitious reports focusing on the American health care system ever undertaken. In the foreword, it noted that the report "addresses quality related issues more broadly, providing a strategic direction for redesigning the health care delivery system of the twenty-first century. Fundamental reform of health care is needed to ensure that all Americans receive care that is safe, effective, patient centered, timely, efficient, and equitable." Words on the opening page—largely written by Berwick—have echoed throughout the health care community for nearly a decade now:

Health care today harms too frequently and routinely fails to deliver its potential benefits. Americans should be able to count on receiving care that meets their needs and is based on the best scientific knowledge. Yet there is strong evidence that this frequently is not the case. Crucial reports from disciplined review bodies document the scale and gravity of the problems. . . . Quality problems are everywhere, affecting many patients. Between the health care we have and the health care we could have lies not just a gap, but a chasm.

The report found that there were massive shortcomings in translating known best practices into common usage. New discoveries, even for treatments for some of the most common chronic diseases, often took many years to be incorporated into use by doctors and hospitals. Far too often, doctors were ignoring or unaware of much better treatments for their patients. Thus, on a widespread scale, patients were not receiving the quality of care that was *known and available*. The failure by hospitals and physician practices to implement newer and more effective treatments was one of the two serious quality shortcomings identified by the committee. The other involved a failure by hospitals and physician practices to use IT to provide better care. The report found that "the current care systems cannot do the job. Trying harder will not work. Changing systems of care will."

The report enunciated four broad goals for transforming the health care system, including better alignment of payment incentives, developing an infrastructure to support evidence-based care, better preparation for the healthcare workforce, and broader use of IT, which the committee noted seemed to have penetrated every corner of American life except health care.

The committee recognized that IT could play a central role in the practice of evidence-based medicine.

Carefully-designed, evidence-based care processes, supported by automated clinical information and decision support systems, offer the greatest promise of achieving the best outcomes from care for chronic conditions [the report stated]. Evidence-based practice guidelines e been developed for many chronic conditions. . . . Yet studies of the quality of care document tremendous variability in practice for many such conditions.

In the current health care system, scientific knowledge about best care is not applied systematically or expeditiously to clinical practice. An average of about 17 years is required for new knowledge generated by randomized controlled trials to be incorporated into practice, and even then practice is highly uneven. . . . The extreme variability in practice in clinical areas in which there is strong scientific evidence and a high degree of expert consensus about best practices indicates that current dissemination efforts fail to reach many clinicians and patients, and that there are insufficient tools and incentives to promote rapid adoption of best practices. The time has come to invest in the creation of a more effective infrastructure for the application of knowledge to health care delivery.

Evidence-based care was best practiced by clinicians with access to computerized Electronic Medical Records that also included a decision support function providing doctors with treatment options and guidelines. Although some clinicians resisted this approach, the reality was that no doctor could possibly keep abreast of all the latest medical advances. A 1998 article in the *Millbank Quarterly* by Mark R. Chassin, MD, detailed the growth in published research from 200 articles in 1975 to more than 30,000 published in 2005. The *Chasm* report stated that "no unaided human being can read, recall, and act effectively on the volume of clinically relevant scientific literature. . . . Weed (2000) has pointed out that to ask an individual practitioner to rely on his or her memory to store and retrieve all the facts relevant to patient care is like asking a travel agent to memorize airline schedules."

A critically important recommendation called for aligning payment methods with quality improvement and in the process, abandoning payment systems that encouraged waste and repetition. For decades, health care had operated on a perverse incentive: Too often, hospitals profit financially when they harm patients. A patient in for surgery would pay a certain amount, but if it so happened that the patient received a staph infection and was forced to remain hospitalized for eight days instead of five, there could be financial benefit to the hospital. The payment system, the *Chasm* report said, was effectively rewarding poor quality, making health care one of the few industries—perhaps the only major sector of the economy—in which payment systems were in no way aligned with quality.

Chasm was embraced by many people throughout health care who agreed with its prescriptive elements, but it received nothing remotely close to the public attention lavished upon *To Err Is Human.*

"I think *To Err Is Human* had been the public call to arms," Berwick reflects. "It's been the one the press could pick up on and use. The *Chasm* report has served the same function, but in a more cloistered side of health care leadership."

The two IOM reports mark a critical juncture in the new quality movement. Together, the reports made the case that American medicine was not only well below the quality level ascribed to it but also, far too often, just plain dangerous. Nonetheless, even in the wake of the IOM reports there were doubters, particularly among physicians. The reports' message was contrary to everything they had ever been taught to believe, contrary to the foundation of the American medical culture. Particularly revealing was a study by researchers from the Harvard School of Public Health and the Kaiser Family Foundation into attitudes of physicians and the public toward the findings in *To Err Is Human.* The study found that doctors were skeptical of the IOM report and did not believe the estimate that medical errors annually killed from 44,000 to 98,000 patients—that they believed it was more on the order of 5,000 per year. Yet the survey also found that more than a third of physicians and four in ten members of the public had experienced a medical error affecting a member of their family or themselves.

By the time this survey had been conducted, Betsy Lehman had been dead for seven years, and the movement toward transparency had begun to take root in a number of major hospitals throughout the country. Increasingly, hospital administrators and physician leaders were coming around to the idea that it was important to disclose errors as a way to learn from them and thus prevent harm in the future. But the overwhelming majority of the doctors in the Harvard/Kaiser study (86 percent) said that errors should be kept private. At the other end of the spectrum were 62 percent of patients who said that errors should be made public.

For those who had yet to join the new quality movement, the most compelling reason to do so was about to be revealed in the form of new data from RAND. During the years after *Chasm,* Beth McGlynn and her colleagues at RAND would publish landmark work on quality, none more crucial than a June 2003 article in the *New England Journal of Medicine* titled "The Quality of Health Care Delivered to Adults in the United States." This was an in-depth national study of adults in twelve metropolitan areas that included a detailed review of medical records and interviews. It may well have been the most comprehensive health care quality study ever done anywhere in the world.

And the central finding was astonishing. The study revealed that American adults received the appropriate recommended care *only about half the time.* This finding was true for adults needing preventive care, acute care, and chronic care. The idea that American adults received the appropriate recommended care only about half the time seemed madness, heresy—absurd on its face. How could this possibly be true?

In the years ahead, disciples of the new quality movement would begin speeches, articles, and classroom discussions citing that single

RAND statistic as an indicator of the quality problem in the United States. Work by McGlynn and her RAND colleagues found that the quality care deficit in the United States is not confined to a particular geographic area nor a particular socioeconomic level. The RAND work, perhaps as surprising as anything else unearthed, shows that *all* Americans are at risk for poor quality care: rich and poor, the highly educated and the uneducated, the well-insured and the uninsured. As McGlynn put it: "Quality of care is a problem nationally, it's a problem in the community where you live and it's a problem for you."

And it is a problem that can be fixed. Much better, safer health care is within our reach. Doctors, nurses, administrators, hospital trustees—men and women in various locations throughout the country—are blazing a new trail. The labors of Don Berwick, Paul Batalden, Lucian Leape; of the Birthday Club and RAND; of Bob Brook and Beth McGlynn; of Janet Corrigan and the IHI, and of all the others committed to improving care, show that converts are out there; men and women who will not rest until health care in America reaches its full quality potential.

5

First, Do No Harm

*"In highly reliable industries there's not one portion
of the organization that's allowed to flounder while
the others thrive. But in health care . . . "*

On the day in 1999 when Rick Shannon was called into the president's office at Allegheny General Hospital, he was already a star. He had risen rapidly through the ranks, from chief medical resident at Beth Israel Hospital in Boston to working under the renowned cardiologist Eugene Brunwald, to training in cardiology at Massachusetts General Hospital. He became associate director of cardiology at Brigham and Women's Hospital in Boston while still in his thirties, and simultaneously served as the chief of cardiology at a Boston Veterans Administration Hospital.

In 1997, when he was just forty-three, Shannon was lured to Allegheny General Hospital in Pittsburgh to serve as chairman of medicine—where he crashed squarely into the quality issue. One day, the CEO of his hospital called him to her office and explained that a public report of cardio-thoracic surgery outcomes would show less than exemplary results for Allegheny; that the results were not as good as their competitors and worse than they might have expected. To complicate matters, the results were going to be released publicly, which would be humiliating for Allegheny General. She explained that this was part of an initiative by the Pittsburgh Regional Health Initiative (PRHI), a private group working with hospitals to improve quality and safety.

Shannon's urgent assignment was to attend a meeting hosted by the PRHI and to defend the honor of Allegheny General. "She wanted me to remind people that these data reflected one of the darkest moments in our history, that our patients were sicker, that they were older, that they had more co-morbidities," Shannon recalls. The point was for Shannon to come up with any explanation he could think of to challenge the new data.

Shannon did not expect that the task would be particularly difficult. He was a gifted speaker with a natural talent for persuasion. The Pittsburgh Regional Health Initiative was led, after all, by a business person, not a physician. The PRHI leader, Paul O'Neill, was CEO of Alcoa, the vast international conglomerate based in Pittsburgh. Alcoa was the largest producer of aluminum products in the world, with nearly 100,000 employees in forty countries. O'Neill was an accomplished business person with a national reputation, but his lack of clinical background gave Shannon a significant edge in any medical discussion. Shannon studied the report searching for "defects in the data, or the data analysis, or the methodology, or misclassification of a case or two—all of which would make a difference. I knew there would be other doctors there, but I knew that I was addressing Mr. O'Neill, and how could he possibly out-duel me on the issue of cardiac surgical outcomes?"

Shannon arrived well-prepared. When the results were presented, it was clear that Allegheny's were worse than anyone else's, yet he launched into skilled, articulate obfuscation, listing ostensible reasons—excuses, really—for why the data weren't quite right. X, y, and z weren't taken into account, these things can be quite complex, and so on and so forth. When he had finished, Rick Shannon thought he had performed quite effectively, but Paul O'Neill had a different view.

"Dr. Shannon," O'Neill said, "thank you for your comments, but you've missed the point."

Shannon was taken aback.

"How so?" he asked.

"We actually aren't here for you to tell us why you had poor results," O'Neill replied. "We're here for you to tell us what you have learned from this and how we can all share in that learning so that we don't ever have to have poor results. We invited you here to understand and to learn from your adverse experiences; not for you to try and justify why they're adverse. We're creating a community of learning here, not a community of blame."

Shannon was caught off guard. *Who is this guy?* he wondered. *What's this all about?*

Paul O'Neill was renowned for his work at Alcoa, where he served as chairman and CEO for twelve years. Not only did he lead the company to new levels of profitability but he took a world-wide organization riddled with safety violations and injuries and made it into the safest industrial corporation in the world. During his tenure, accidents that resulted in days lost from work went from 1.86 per 100 employees down to 0.2. This he accomplished in a company employing 100,000-plus people who conducted highly dangerous operations in dozens of nations around the world; in some plants, they handled metals at 2,000 degrees.

In 1997, O'Neill was among a group of civic, business, and health care leaders in western Pennsylvania working to attract capital investment to the area while at the same time improving the quality of life. They identified health care as a key improvement target and thus established the Pittsburgh Regional Health Initiative as an independent body to promote quality and safety while controlling costs. O'Neill believed that the industrial techniques he had employed so successfully at Alcoa would translate well into health care. PRHI, which would soon grow to a consortium of forty-three western Pennsylvania hospitals, started in 1997 with clear goals: "Zero hospital-acquired infections. Zero medication errors. The world's best patient outcomes in five clinical areas: cardiac surgery; obstetrical care for mother and child; orthopedic surgery of hip and knee; diabetes; and depression." The goal was "perfect care for every patient."

This was revolutionary stuff at the time. O'Neill and the PRHI were years ahead of the curve; they actively focused on the safety/quality issue a full two years before the publication of *To Err Is Human*.

The day after the meeting, O'Neill called Shannon and invited him to lunch, where he tried to enlist Shannon in the PRHI campaign. "He sat me down," Shannon recalls, "and said, 'Listen, I can tell from the way you presented yourself that you have all the right instincts to be a leader in this. I want you to join me. I want you to be actively engaged in this. I want to teach you what I know about this. I want you to understand, as I do, what the opportunity is, because I think you could really help us with this.'"

O'Neill told Shannon about his safety approach at Alcoa and his use of principles from the Toyota Production System. The key to improvement, he told Shannon, was leadership, and O'Neill invited Shannon to help provide some of the much needed leadership in Pittsburgh. To Paul O'Neill, the term *leadership* was not some vaguely defined concept. In fact, he had a precise definition of the term, which he shared with Shannon:

> A real leader creates the culture where it's possible for people to say yes to three propositions every day without reservation: I'm treated with dignity and respect by everyone I encounter every day without regard to my job title or educational attainment or my race or my ethnicity or my gender or any other distinguishing characteristic. Number two, I'm given the things I need—education, tools, training, encouragement so I can make a contribution that gives meaning to my life. And third, I'm recognized for what I do.

The first task of leadership, said O'Neill, is to create this sort of environment. The second task is for a leader "to accept responsibility for everything that goes wrong in the organization—no one else is responsible for anything gone wrong. Because at the end of the day in most organizations the CEO has the ability to create a situation where things don't go wrong."

This was all brand new to Rick Shannon. He had, to that point in his career, been a traditionalist. He played by the standard rules of medicine, had performed exceptionally well, and had risen steadily through the ranks. At that point—1999—the new quality movement was, depending upon how one calculates, anywhere from twelve to thirty years old. Yet Shannon, like most clinicians throughout the United States, was largely unaware of it. He may have glanced at a Lucian Leape article along the way, but the quality movement was not a blip on his radar. Ironically, Shannon knew Don Berwick, who had been an attending when Shannon trained at the Brigham in Boston, but Shannon had no idea that Berwick had gone on to become one of the world's quality leaders (later, when Shannon was deeply immersed in quality work himself, he would describe Berwick as the movement's "intellectual driving force").

"Until my chance meeting with Paul O'Neill I was a basic scientist with no interest, training, or experience whatsoever in what I would call outcomes research," he says. "Nor did I have interest, training, or any idea about the magnitude of what the current condition, characterized by unsafe conditions, really meant to the health care system."

But he was fascinated by O'Neill's pitch at lunch and impressed with O'Neill's seriousness of purpose. He was also intrigued by the possibility of applying Alcoa-type techniques to health care. Most of all, Shannon liked the idea of working with cardiologists from other hospitals in western Pennsylvania to pool brain power and learn from one another. That approach, which was what PRHI was all about, seemed to Shannon to be something that could benefit patients, physicians, the entire community.

After his lunch with O'Neill, Shannon met with Connie Cibrone, the Allegheny CEO, explained what he and O'Neill had discussed, and told her that he was interested in working with O'Neill and the PRHI. There was a hitch, though, he told her. O'Neill was a believer in transparency and he wanted the hospitals to disclose a variety of data publicly. She was surprised. She wondered aloud why he would want to do that. It seemed to her, she told Shannon, that it made no sense for a hospital to disclose bad news. Shannon understood her point of view, of course, and believed it made perfect sense. He decided to go to PRHI meetings and deal with the transparency issue if it was raised. But he did not actually believe there would be disclosure of poor outcomes: None of the forty-three hospitals involved in the PRHI would agree to that, so he wasn't particularly concerned.

But the issue was raised at one of the first PRHI sessions when O'Neill argued that the press should be allowed to attend meetings. This notion was met with vehement opposition from just about everybody in the room. Hospital officials—doctors, nurses, administrators—did not want to share their most intimate and embarrassing secrets about errors only to have the stories plastered across the front page of the newspapers.

But O'Neill thought it made perfect sense to allow the press in the room. "Our job is to educate the press and the public how to understand these things gone wrong," he said. "You can't conceal it from them. You are far better off educating them about it, inviting them in, than you are letting them try to write about it on their own."

To Shannon and the other providers the idea was not only absurd but potentially self-destructive. When Shannon explained the situation to his CEO, she was adamant—there was no way Allegheny would participate. Shannon took this message to O'Neill hoping he would reconsider his position. "I'm really captivated by the notions that you espouse," he told O'Neill, "but I'm going to have a problem if the press is in the room. That's my marching order. I work for my CEO. My CEO says, 'No deal if the press is there.'"

O'Neill considered this and then had a suggestion. How about this, he said: We invite the press into the meetings, but for the next six months they cannot write any stories. The idea would be to educate them, to get them to see the bigger picture and understand the struggle for quality and safety: "If we're going to create a community of learning where safety becomes a precondition, and we're going to create a community where there are no trade secrets about who does what well, then the press has to be part of that agreement," O'Neill told Shannon. "And so, I'll meet with the members of the press. I'll invite them in and I will say they are capable of taking notes. I will say that for a period of time this must be kept here as they learn."

And it worked. O'Neill had enough influence in the city—based not only on his success at Alcoa but on his many civic and charitable efforts as well—that the press was willing to go along. Every other week at the PRHI meetings there were the reporters "listening to this man educate a group of people about what it meant to commit in an unfailing way to having the safest health care system in the region. It was remarkable. He had such sway over every-body in that room."

And over Rick Shannon, as well. Shannon had heard about the depth of O'Neill's commitment to safety when he first went to Alcoa for a meeting with members of the PRHI. He met others who, upon arriving, had been given a certificate for a free cup of coffee for wearing their seat belts as they pulled into the parking lot.

> I walk into the Alcoa corporate headquarters, into this meeting room and there was a group of people and Paul O'Neill says, "I want every-one to be aware of where the fire exits are. And what the fastest route of evacuation is in event of an emergency." I'm thinking, "What is this guy talking about?" . . . So, when you talk about walking the walk, from the moment I entered the place, there was a culture of safety—not a safety officer—safety was *everybody's* business. Just seeing that had an enormous impact upon me. In health care, what we do is set up this silo that says—you're the patient safety officer. That means we must be doing safety—because we've got someone called the patient safety officer.

PRHI created a course called Perfecting Patient Care, which served as an introduction to the principles of the Toyota Production System specifically and industrial quality techniques generally. As part of the course, they read a case study of the Toyota plant in Georgetown, Ken-tucky, and Shannon later had a chance to visit the plant. "Everything about this manufacturing plant was visual," he says, recalling a series of placards portraying the entire manufacturing process.

> I spent a lot of time watching the worker responsible for placing the left front seat into the Camry. The concept was to examine both the reliability and the precision and specification with which he did the work. I watched this guy bolt the seat in. Left front lug nut first; right

front lug nut; left rear; right rear. The same way every time all in about five seconds. . . . The precision with which they did this, the specification as to sequencing and timing and expected outcome were an extraordinary sight to see.

As he observed the precision of the Toyota process, Shannon had visions of nurses rummaging through drawers filled with various medications, some of which in color, size, and even name, could easily be confused, especially by a tired, overworked nurse at the end of a shift. *Why*, Shannon wondered, *do I have eighteen ampicillin pills in the drawer, and why do they never arrive at eight o'clock when the order is written? Why, sometimes, does the nurse go there and there are none? Why, sometimes, does she put her hand in the wrong drawer for the patient's medicine? And what about the look-alike medications?*

"Watching that process was exactly like watching medication delivery," Shannon recalls, "except one was highly precise and very reliable and the other was total chaos." The Toyota system handed the worker only the bolt he needed, eliminating the possibility of human error. A car manufacturing facility had a better system to distribute bolts than his hospital had to distribute medication: "The fact that he never had more than the next lug nut available to him taught me about their supply chain—which wasn't that he had a bucket full of lug nuts there that he took; it was—*we know how many we need, and we get them when we need them.* Everything was done one by one to a specific outcome, with a specific precision, that, if it wasn't met, the entire assembly line stopped."

Rick Shannon grew increasingly attracted to the PRHI approach and Paul O'Neill's philosophy that industrial quality techniques could be used effectively in health care. As he worked with physicians from a dozen other western Pennsylvania hospitals on improving quality and safety in cardiac surgery, Shannon found that the group had become a community united in the pursuit of learning—in most cases, from one another's mistakes. When they gathered for private meetings, each hospital cardiology department would bare its soul, revealing what had gone wrong. Doctors would arrive at the meetings clenching thick files—medical records of patients who had died under their care. This was not easy to do. There was in fact something quite solemn about this exercise, for these were men and women who cared deeply about their patients and who worked extraordinarily hard seeking to cure them. Sometimes mistakes were made. In the past, for the most part, those mistakes were kept extremely quiet within each individual institution. The culture of medicine had long favored silence and secrecy in such matters, but in Pittsburgh that was changing.

On Thursday, October 16, 2002, one of Allegheny General's infection control staff members approached Rick Shannon with a serious problem. She thought that one of the bronchoscopes might be contaminated and that two patients might have been exposed, but she was uncertain what had caused the contamination. (A bronchoscope is a thin tube used to explore the interior of the upper airway and lungs and is typically inserted through the patient's nose or mouth.) "This was all hush-hush," recalls Shannon. "No one was supposed to know about it."

There was some history to the problem, Shannon knew. Back in July, several ICU patients had been afflicted with Pseudomonas bacterial infections. Pseudomonas, though a common bacterium in humans, generally causes harm only when a patient is already weakened by illness. Among patients suffering from cancer, AIDS, or diabetes, for example, the mortality rate from those infected with Pseudomonas was 50 percent. But back in the summer, the problem had been quickly solved by standard infection protection measures. Now, in October, the problem appeared to have returned. Several ICU patients were infected with a strain of Pseudomonas resistant to traditional antibiotics.

On October 11, the hospital pulled the surgical intensive care unit's bronchoscope for testing. Four days later, tests revealed that resistant Pseudomonas were growing from cultures taken from the bronchoscope. That triggered testing of other bronchoscopes, two of which showed they were also contaminated with a similar strain found in the patients.

First, Shannon wanted to make sure that no other patient was exposed to the bronchoscopes. He ordered all tests scheduled for the next day—Friday—cancelled. This seemed to him a no-brainer because they were elective procedures that could easily be rescheduled for the following week. But the Allegheny chief operating officer (COO) pushed back. A dozen procedures should not be summarily cancelled, he argued. Shannon spoke to the COO: "We can schedule these cases for Monday," he said, "because by Monday, working together, we can figure out what's wrong here. But if you run the risk of exposing one more human being to what is yet an undetermined point source of a contaminated piece of equipment, I'll resign." The cases were postponed.

Friday afternoon around 2:00 P.M., Allegheny CEO Connie Cibrone called Shannon and assigned him to lead an investigation into the root cause of the infections and to report back on a remedy that would prevent it from happening in the future. Shannon convened a team of twelve people to work with him on various parts of the investigation. During the next forty hours, from Friday afternoon until Sunday morning, Rick Shannon did not leave the hospital. By late Friday night, the cause had not yet been discovered, but Shannon did learn that it was not just two patients who had been infected; it was sixteen. Throughout much of Saturday afternoon, while his team continued trying to solve the puzzle, Shannon felt compelled to inform the doctors about the patients infected, as well as the patients themselves.

Also on Saturday, the infection control group at Allegheny informed Shannon that Johns Hopkins had faced a similar problem just a few months earlier. The infection team contacted their counterparts at Hopkins to discuss the matter. Hopkins had contacted all patients who had been tested by the bronchoscopes for six weeks prior to the problem and asked them to come in for examination. Shannon and the team decided to double that and call in the 586 patients who had been to Allegheny for a bronchoscope in the past three months. A system was set up to test every one of the patients (85 percent of those patients eventually came in for testing, and none had been infected).

On Saturday, one of the sixteen infected patients died. The sense of urgency grew. That day, Shannon's team contacted the Centers for Disease Control (CDC) to determine whether they had seen similar problems, and they had. Some of the problems had been related to the disinfectant used to sterilize the bronchoscopes. At Allegheny, they used periacetic acid to cleanse the scope. It was fast—requiring an hour to disinfect—and effective, and it was certainly preferable to using the gas sterilization method which, although flawless, took twenty-four hours.

By Sunday, thanks to their own diligence and guidance from Hopkins and CDC, the mystery appeared to be solved. After every use a scope would be placed in the cleaning machine and treated with acid that killed all germs in the scope. This was followed by four rinse cycles during which tap water passed through a biological filter that, in theory at least, filtered out all bacteria. The problem, they discovered, was that over time the biological filter broke down and lost its effectiveness, allowing bacteria to pass through into the water. What they thought was a procedure to disinfect a bronchoscope was actually contaminating it. In retrospect, canceling the procedures scheduled for Friday proved quite fortunate, for any number of those patients might also have become infected.

During his learning process with PRHI, Shannon had come to believe in transparency. He saw that hiding mistakes was harmful to patients and that revealing them enabled the entire medical community to learn. Sunday afternoon, Shannon met with the CEO and chairman of the board of trustees and suggested that on Monday it would be appropriate to disclose publicly what had happened. This disclosure would send a clear signal that Allegheny was open and honest with patients and prospective patients, and it would encourage other hospitals to examine comparable machinery to head off possible problems. If the PRHI mission of community learning meant anything, this was the time to test it. The hospital communications staff strenuously objected to disclosure. The board chairman held a similar view. But Shannon argued that the news would inevitably leak out to the press. When the folks at Johns Hopkins faced a similar situation a few months earlier, they did not disclose it publicly, but the press got wind of it anyway. In Allegheny General's case, the news would most certainly leak to the press because the patient death Saturday had been reported to the county coroner. "We either get in front of this and acknowledge that we have a problem and that we're sharing what we've learned, or we are really going to look bad," Shannon said. He added that they had discovered something of real clinical value: The quicker sterilization method was not always reliable and could even harm patients. *We have an obligation,* he argued, *to get that information out there as fast as possible to as many hospitals as possible to reduce the chances of it happening to any other human being.* "When we make a mistake the public expects us to acknowledge it and take steps to make sure it never happens again," Shannon argued. The discussion dragged on throughout the rest of Sunday night without resolution.

The next day, all Allegheny bronchoscopes were removed from service and replaced by new instruments. The hospital adopted a policy of using a new, more reliable method of disinfecting. On a substantive level, the matter could hardly have been handled much better: The patients affected were promptly notified, as were their doctors; the source of the infections was discovered and contained and new equipment—with better disinfectant techniques—was put into service. And all this was achieved in one weekend.

But on Monday, the issue of how to deal with the matter publicly, or whether to do so, seemed no closer to resolution. At one point, someone in the administration made a comment that triggered an idea from Shannon.

"We don't think we can go out there alone," the administrator said. Shannon seized on the word *alone*. What if, he suggested, we could get the Pittsburgh Regional Health Initiative to stand with us? Why don't we call the county health commissioner, inform him, and see whether he'll stand with us?

Shannon contacted Bruce Dixon, the county health commissioner, and explained the situation and Dickson immediately saw the advantage in making the story public to help other hospitals head off similar problems. He said he would definitely support Allegheny in their disclosure. Paul O'Neill, who had left Alcoa to become treasury secretary, also fully supported disclosure and said he was sure the leadership of PRHI would stand with Allegheny leaders publicly. Allegheny officials agreed to make the announcement, and did so with visible support from the county health commissioner and representatives from PRHI. In fact, PRHI pledged to convene a regional meeting of the forty-three PRHI hospitals and educate everyone about the case in an effort to head it off from happening anywhere else.

At a press conference that afternoon—flanked by PRHI officials and the county health commissioner—Shannon explained what had occurred since the discovery of the problem Friday. They made a public offer to work with any other health care organizations discovering a comparable problem.

Rather than sensationalize the Allegheny problem and demonize the hospital in the process, the press played the story straight—absent the scolding attitude that might have been common elsewhere. Perhaps the press had been influenced by the idea that identifying defects enables others to prevent or fix them elsewhere—that the process was about a community learning together to improve the quality of care. If so, it was to the credit of the Pittsburgh media. Little more than a month later, the *Post-Gazette* followed up with a detailed article focused on the lessons learned from the incident that might benefit other hospitals and patients. An article in the newspaper the following year lauded Shannon's actions in the case:

> When Allegheny General Hospital found itself under public scrutiny from a bacterial outbreak that killed a patient, the institution had the choice of clamming up reflexively or volunteering information on what problems had occurred.
>
> To Dr. Richard Shannon, the hospital's chief of medicine since 1997, that was no choice at all. He won praise for the hospital's forthright handling of an investigation and public attention in the months after the October 2002 spread of Pseudomonas bacteria to 16 patients, one of whom died.
>
> Shannon, 48, a cardiologist who was a longtime faculty member at Harvard Medical School before coming to Pittsburgh, believes his profession is too often its own worst enemy for tolerating or covering up errors.
>
> "We felt very strongly that the public at large should be apprised of the problem, in the event that people had questions or concerns we could help them with."

In 2002, when Paul O'Neill left the Treasury Department and returned to Pittsburgh, Shannon was exultant. "Here returns the hero," he thought. "Now he had such stature that it was really the opportunity in Pittsburgh to go deep and to really create a national demonstration." O'Neill told him: "I'm going to devote myself to this.

We're going to make Pittsburgh great. We're going to have the nation come and see us."

Shannon was thrilled, for this was the type of goal that he believed O'Neill's leadership could help achieve. "We've got a lot of traction here and I think it's time that we start to do something bold," he replied. Shannon was, of course, preaching to the choir. O'Neill returned to Pittsburgh with the concept that "in a very short period of time he want[ed] to transform the region," recalls Shannon. "If there's one thing I would say about Paul O'Neill—he is not a patient man." He wanted results and he wanted them quickly, and he knew from his experience at Alcoa that rapid progress was eminently possible.

Back in Pittsburgh, however, O'Neill found the pace of change too slow. There were islands of excellence, to be sure, but they seemed to exist in a sea of chaos. In institutions such as Shannon's, there was progress in one unit but not in others; and some hospitals were progressing incrementally, others not at all. Paul O'Neill was not a man interested in plodding, incremental change. He said that if Pittsburgh was to be great—a model for the country—then decisive action was required. It was the spring of 2003 when O'Neill said that he wanted to jump-start the PRHI initiative by asking "every hospital in this region to declare, publicly, a goal of eliminating certain classes of hospital-acquired infections and to give us a date of when they're going to do it."

This was as bold and aggressive as it got in American health care at the time. Nothing like this had ever been attempted before, certainly not on as large a scale as O'Neill was proposing. And for good reason: Hospital administrators and most physician leaders thought it unwise; unwise because they believed it was not attainable and because inevitable failure would trigger ridicule from colleagues and the press. This was the mindset that believed unshakably in the proposition that complications in medicine were inevitable; complications—mistakes, really—were a cost of doing business. Perhaps

O'Neill expected the hospitals to embrace his goal with enthusiasm. Perhaps he expected that they would feel they had no choice. But his bold aspiration was not widely shared. Behind the scenes grumbling came from hospital leaders who wanted to know why Paul O'Neill was stomping on their turf and telling them what to do.

"There were a lot of misgivings," recalls Shannon. "A lot of people said, 'Who is Paul O'Neill to set the health care agenda?' Many people said he didn't understand. Others said it's just not possible and others were just offended he was getting so much attention." But Shannon made a headlong commitment to O'Neill's approach. "I had really become a believer that we could apply methods from reliable industries and I was fully engaged. I believed we should dare to be great and not creep up on it in some reluctant fashion."

He went back to Allegheny and told the hospital leadership about the goal O'Neill had proposed. The section chiefs and hospital administration were clearly uncomfortable with O'Neill's approach and wanted to set a more modest target. How about this, they said, we'll set a goal of reducing infections by, say, 10 percent, or 15 percent. That way, they would be participating in the effort but with a much more reasonable goal. They took this position not because they were opposed to improvement or weren't excellent doctors and administrators; rather, like so many people in health care, they believed that these infections were inevitable and that there was only so much that could be done. Shannon understood this, but knew the incremental approach was exactly what O'Neill was trying to avoid.

"How about this," he suggested to the CEO. "You declare some modest goal on behalf of the organization—'we're going to reduce infections by ten percent over the next two years,' or whatever you want to decide . . . and I'm going to take the two units that I control, and I'm going to eliminate central line infections in ninety days, and then I'm going to show you how I did it."

The reaction around the table was predictable: *Are you crazy? Why would you do that?* But to her credit, CEO Connie Cibrone gave Shannon the go-ahead to try.

At the beginning, Shannon knew he needed the support and enthusiasm of the doctors and nurses who worked in the intensive care units (ICUs). To have any chance at success, the clinical staff had to see the mission clearly and believe in it wholeheartedly. Any sense that this was an imposed goal from leadership forced down upon the workers from above would guarantee failure. He gathered the nurses together first and said, "We're going to do something here that no one else has ever done. Our goal is to make this the safest ICU for any human being to be in, in America."

Although the nursing staff liked Shannon's enthusiasm, there was some hesitation, an instinctive reaction that the goal, while noble, was impossible to achieve. The nurses, after all, had not had a fraction of Shannon's exposure to quality improvement techniques; they had not heard O'Neill preach his quality gospel; and they had not taken the PRHI course Shannon had taken (Perfecting Patient Care). As a result, there wasn't the level of buy-in Shannon felt was needed to make the program work.

And then the turning point came, as it so often does in medicine, with a tragic event.

Rick Shannon had cared for a particular patient—we'll call him Mr. Williams—for a number of years. Mr. Williams was in his late fifties and his heart disease had progressively worsened over time until the point more than two years earlier when Shannon had placed him on the list for a heart transplant.

In July 2003, just as Shannon was trying to launch his safety initiative, he received a call from a cardiologist caring for Mr. Williams saying that the patient was having difficulty. Since Mr. Williams lived some distance from Pittsburgh, the cardiologist had him admitted to a local hospital where he was given dobutamine to stimulate his cardiac output. The drug was administered intravenously and served to strengthen Mr. Williams's weakening heart. The fact that dobutamine was administered also moved Mr. Williams up the heart priority list from status 2 to status 1, a significant advancement that put him near the front of the line for an available heart.

After waiting for two and a half years for a heart, Mr. Williams was very close, but soon after the dobutamine was administered, the cardiologist called Shannon with troubling news. Mr. Williams had developed bacterimia (the presence of bacteria in the bloodstream) and it appeared the source was the IV catheter. Mr. Williams was transferred to Rick Shannon's ICU, but now that a powerful infection had rendered the patient gravely ill, he was removed from the transplant list, too sick to undergo surgery for a new heart.

Thirteen days later, Mr. Williams died. Shannon sat with Mr. Williams's wife and daughters and did his best to explain what had happened. The family was in disbelief. One of his daughters said to Shannon: "You mean after all this time and all this hope and all this work, my father died from an *IV infection?*"

"Yes," Shannon replied, "your father died from an IV infection."

An entirely preventable IV infection—though he did not say that. Shannon and the two principle nurses who had cared for Mr. Williams were deeply shaken. As experienced clinical professionals in an ICU unit, they were accustomed to dire cases, but here was a man on the verge of gaining new life and he was killed by an infection given to him in a hospital.

"The nurses who were taking care of this man were in tears. This wasn't a statistic. It was a human being—*a human being.* They also saw this paradox of how we had worked so hard to provide this man with the highest technological care, and it was totally undone by what I was arguing was a preventable error."

The loss of Mr. Williams spurred the clinical staff forward. His pre-cipitous decline—from such hope one day to death weeks later—had stunned them. Shannon could see that the nurses on his unit, in particular, were absolutely ready for change, but that did not yet ap-pear to be the case with the physicians. Shannon knew the physician culture. He knew for certain that trying to force anything down their throats was doomed to failure. He wanted to appeal to their intel-lect, but he also believed he needed to inject humanity into it as well. He wanted to translate the statistics of central line infections into the *human reality* of central line infections; from "some epidemi-ological statistic, five point one infections per thousand line days, into real, human stories—faces, names, consequences."

Shannon went back into the files and pulled records for all pa-tients who had suffered a central line infection during the past year. The record included the name of the attending physician in each case. Shannon met privately with each doctor to, as he put it, "de-code the data"; that is, use the data and facts of the case to paint a human portrait. There was real concern among the doctors that Shannon was in possession of this data—that he knew about the mistakes at all. He assured them that this was not a blame game, but rather that he wanted them to have the information so that they would know what needed to be improved. With the nurses and doc-tors now both ready to strive for change, the question became: Change *what,* exactly? And the answer wasn't at all clear.

If step one in the process was decoding the data, step two was ob-servation. Shannon spent weeks observing the insertion of central lines. What he saw was remarkable: Some doctors wore masks and caps, some didn't; some wore gowns, some didn't; some used special sterile drapes, some didn't; some used one form of disinfectant, others didn't. On top of all this, five different types of catheter were being used. "We found fifty or sixty permutations of the way this was done. That creates such background chaos that *no one knows what the right way to do it is."* It was, recalls Shannon, "like making an automobile a new way every time you make one."

Once it was clear to Shannon that there was no uniformity—nothing approaching a best practice or standard work—he gathered the team together and said their mission was to figure out the best practice for each and every step of the process. "Let's all agree there's one way to do this," he said. This was the notion of standard work so crucial in industrial quality; the idea that there is a best way to perform any procedure; a *correct* way; a *safe* way; that variation is the enemy and leads to defects.

Shannon did not make the mistake of prescribing the correct way to insert a line. He left that to the doctors and nurses who were actually doing the work. A solution imposed from above would be no solution at all. If the front-line clinicians developed a best practice by assembling their collective wisdom and experience to identify the right method, they were much more likely to adhere to its standards. Shannon stayed involved every step of the way, making it clear this was his priority.

After several weeks of work, the team had come up with an approach: Doctors would wear masks and caps. They would wear gowns. They agreed on one disinfectant. They agreed that the patient would have to be draped—a protective, sterile field around the point of insertion (usually in the neck). They agreed on a precise order and what the nurse would do and what the doctor would do. They identified a specific type of catheter they would use. At the end of the process, the team had identified a crystal clear standard of work and anyone who didn't follow the standard work would be called on it by nurses or other physicians.

However, the team quickly saw that they had no standard way of maintaining the line and keeping the catheter sterile. Thus they went through the same process and developed a standard process for maintaining the line.

Shannon felt the process was right. They had a new way of doing the work—"not necessarily the perfect way," he says. "One of the enemies of quality improvement is this notion that you've got to get it perfect. What you've got to do is change it and test whether it works. If you wait for perfection, it's never going to happen." It wasn't exactly a randomized double-blind scientific study, but it was nonetheless a form of evidence-based care: Each member of the clinical team brought their evidentiary experience to creating a new process. They did not try just one rigid method but adapted their approach as experience taught them how to improve it. He realized that going forward it would be important to place every episode of infection under the microscope, figuratively as well as literally. He and the team committed to getting at the root cause of an infection whenever it occurred, and without delay.

> Historically, when an infection occurred, it would typically be recognized and reported three to six months after it happened. Under those circumstances, sitting in a meeting of quality assurance people, there would be absolutely no way anybody could figure out what happened. And this leads to what I call the *myth of inevitability.* If six months after the fact you're sitting in a room and somebody says, "Why'd that guy get infected?" everyone goes, "Gee, I don't know." It becomes an act of God. . . . Once it becomes inevitable, you lose all sense of responsibility.

Going forward, in any case where there was a potential central line infection (even before it was diagnosed as such), Shannon convened a meeting of all hospital personnel—from doctors to dieticians—who had been involved with the patient. The purpose of the meeting was not to assess blame but to try to learn what happened—valuable information that could help improve the process and prevent infections in the future.

In one case, a patient's catheter was twisted and failed to work. It was the middle of the night and the resident was uncomfortable inserting a new catheter. She spoke with a pulmonary fellow who advised her to place a wire in the catheter and straighten it out. Rewiring catheters was standard practice in medicine, yet after the patient had undergone the procedure the next morning bacteria was discovered in the blood—bacteria identical to that found in the catheter. Shannon recalled:

> The next day, when we had the root cause analysis, I got all the people together, and I said, "Now tell me, the last day or two, what's going on here that might have contributed to this?" And the nurse from that evening said, "Well, two nights ago the catheter kinked; we had a real problem. The patient needed the medication. We didn't know what to do. The resident called the fellow who said to rewire it." And the resident said, "Yeah, I called the fellow. I was worried. I didn't feel comfortable putting lines in myself. I thought the fellow might come in and we could do it together; but the fellow said I should just do this. I didn't quite think it was the right thing to do, but the guy's blood pressure was low, I did my best."
>
> I said, "Very good. Your job was to get the patient through the night; and to make sure this worked properly. It seems to me that what we did was a workaround. What the patient needed, really, was a new catheter. That it was one o'clock in the morning shouldn't matter, we're an intensive care unit. What we should say is that in our unit we don't rewire catheters.
>
> And then I talked to the pulmonary fellow—I said, "You know, what happened the other night was a call for help. The next time you get a call for help, you get your butt out of bed and you get in here and you help. That's your job."
>
> So the learning was, *we're not going to deal with kinked catheters.* We're going to replace them. And anybody who doesn't feel comfortable

doing so is going to activate a help chain. And the help chain needs to respond. That was a classic example. No written note about what happened. No way six months later you could have figured out what happened. And it otherwise would have gone into the bucket of inevitable. *Bad luck. Unavoidable. We did our best.* Instead, we had stumbled upon a new practice, which said we don't rewire catheters here, we replace them. Each one of the infections that we observed generated that kind of immediate learning.

In other words, by closely studying defects and mistakes—precisely what Paul O'Neill had said he wanted to do the first time he met Rick Shannon—Shannon's team was learning critically important lessons.

"My Toyota experience taught me that you investigate any problem immediately down to its root cause," he says. Once you learn the cause, you work on fixing the problem. By subjecting every infection to intensive scrutiny to determine the root cause, Shannon made some surprising discoveries. In one case, a patient with a picc catheter in the arm developed a line infection, but no one could determine the cause. After gathering information from everybody who had had anything to do with the patient, the key came from an environmental services employee, a person who cleaned the rooms. Shannon asked her whether she had seen anything amiss. In fact, she had. She said she saw an ambu bag—which helps patients breathe when they are not on a ventilator—lying atop the patient's catheter. A used ambu bag contains secretions from a patient's breathing and thus plentiful bacteria.

"When I clean these rooms, I find those bags everywhere," she told Shannon. "When I come in the morning, I find them under the patient's pillow. I find them under the patient's sheets, next to the urinal. I found one laying on top of this person's catheter."

It was clear to Shannon that this was the likely cause of the infection. Shannon thanked the woman and she offered some advice: "If I were you, Dr. Shannon, I'd go to Home Depot and I'd get a couple of those hooks, and I would just say, 'The ambu bag belongs here.'" And that is precisely what Shannon did; he bought two dozen hooks from Home Depot, screwed them into the wall, and made it clear that used ambu bags should be stored on the hooks. Total cost of hooks: $12.

Every event such as this added to the body of knowledge that Shannon and his team accumulated: "Each time that you eliminate one of these defects, you dramatically reduce the risk of any one thing propagating into an error," he notes. "We standardized the way we perform the lines. We standardized the way we take care of the lines. Then every time there's a problem, we identify a defect that may have led to it. Each one of those defects leads to what we call a countermeasure where we take lessons and embed them into the work."

After ninety days, the results were clear: There had not been a single central line infection in either of Shannon's units. His team was exultant. To celebrate, Shannon bought Chinese food for a team lunch that included the doctors, nurses, housekeepers, dieticians, and nurses' aides—*everyone*. Over lunch, people talked about what they had learned and offered ideas for improvement. "There was such pride," says Shannon, "because they were now working in the safest units in the hospital."

Looking back over the years he worked at Allegheny, Shannon recalls that the year before he began the quality improvement efforts there were forty-nine central line infections in his units. During the first year of his work there were six; then, because of a change in technology, eleven the next year. The year after that, there were two; and then, the ultimate confirmation of the work he and his team had done, the units went twenty-four months (and counting) without a single infection. He says of the medical staff in the units: "They won't tolerate a central line infection. That's their attitude now."

Shannon found that one of the most difficult aspects of quality improvement is transferring learning to other clinical areas:

> One of the frustrations in all this was the fact that within an organization you could have these outstanding results and next door, what would be considered mediocre results. Part of that is the absence of physician leadership there that says, "I refuse to live this way." . . . Part of it is organizational leadership that says, "We're willing to accept excellence in one area and mediocrity in another."
>
> At Toyota they don't say the tire guys are the best and the guys who put on the mufflers are just average. At Alcoa, they don't have one business unit that's good and another business unit that's bad. In highly reliable industries there's not one portion of the organization that's allowed to flounder while the others thrive. But in health care . . .

While Shannon and his team were flourishing, O'Neill's initiative had began to weaken. The pushback from hospitals grew too intense. It became clear to O'Neill that the hospitals were not willing to be as aggressive as he thought they should be. He resigned from the board at the University of Pittsburgh Medical Center. Shannon regretted seeing the hospitals and O'Neill part ways. He recognized that O'Neill had pushed very hard, but Shannon believed in what O'Neill was striving for—believed it was the right course.

In October 2006, Shannon left Allegheny General for a position as chief of medicine at the University of Pennsylvania Hospital in Philadelphia. Before his departure, the *Post-Gazette* published an editorial praising his work. One way to measure Shannon's impact in Pittsburgh is to ask this question: How often do major newspapers editorialize when a physician moves from one city to another?

At the University of Pennsylvania in Philadelphia, Shannon is hoping to build on the work he started at Allegheny. The main difference from his work in Pittsburgh is that at Penn, he says, "I'm not going to train a unit. I'm going to train *everyone* in the Department of Medicine." He also declared in his state of the department address in September 2007 the Department of Medicine's goal "to eliminate these unsafe conditions embedded in central line infections, ventilator-associated pneumonias, and methicillin resistant staph (MRSA) infections." At the beginning of 2008, Shannon inaugurated a quality improvement effort in the Penn ICU and oncology units to eliminate infections. His plan was to work in those locations for six months, then rapidly spread the work throughout the hospital.

At Penn, he is also planning to take his work to a significantly higher level by collaborating with economists at the Wharton School to conduct an indepth economic analysis of how to increase safety and quality while removing waste and driving down costs.

Rick Shannon believes that within five years the American health care delivery system will be significantly transformed. He envisions the elimination of most hospital-acquired infections. He sees a safer system; a system where waste is reduced and costs better controlled.

When he scans the health care landscape these days, he sees the pioneers of the new quality movement along with a relatively small yet hardy band of practitioners like him committed to and acting on serious change. In the time he has been working on quality and safety issues, Shannon has seen the ranks of those interested in the work grow exponentially. What is needed now, he says, is for those interested clinicians and administrators and others to elevate from interest to commitment.

6

The Cincinnati
Children's Triumvirate:
Uma Kotagal, Jim Anderson, Lee Carter

"We will be the best at getting better."

The journey toward Cincinnati Children's Hospital winning the 2006 American Hospital Association-McKesson Quest for Quality Prize began thirty-one years earlier, on July 1, 1975, when Dr. Uma Kotagal began her fellowship in neonatal physiology at Cincinnati Children's. Twenty-seven-year-old Dr. Kotagal was a striking combination of flowing black hair, piercing gaze, no-nonsense manner, brilliant clinical mind, and fierce commitment to patients. Originally from Bombay, the younng doctor was impossible not to notice. Fellows, by tradition and, typically, inclination, readily deferred to their seniors, the wise men from whom they learned. Dr. Kotagal was perfectly happy to do this when she thought it appropriate, but she was also perfectly willing to complain about the system and the quality of patient care when she felt *that* was warranted. Uma Kotagal and the idea of standing on ceremony for the sake of appearance never quite meshed.

Through the years, and eventually decades, during which she would move to lead the quality improvement work at Cincinnati Children's, Dr. Kotagal would be described in many ways—visionary, relentless, demanding, brilliant—("She punches hard," the CEO would later say of her). During all that time, through many ups and downs, through periods when she sought to revolutionize care, she never lost sight of why she was doing it all. She wanted to improve care for children. It was just that simple—and just that immensely, hugely complicated.

During her fellowship at Cincinnati Children's in the mid-1970s, Uma Kotagal became bothered by the imbalance she saw between research and patient care. It was obvious to her that research was highly valued and patient care less so, *much* less so, she thought. In years past, researchers at Cincinnati Children's had discovered the Sabin oral polio vaccine and a life-saving surfactant preparation for premature babies. Success in research brought professional distinction, sometimes renown, and thus attracted many talented young doctors and PhDs.

Young Dr. Kotagal was all for excellence in research, but as she looked around at the hospital, she wasn't really seeing *clinical* excellence. The reality of care didn't seem to match the vaunted reputation of the hospital. There was a huge gap between research and figuring out how to apply existing knowledge at the bedside. This was the first of countless heretical thoughts Uma Kotagal would entertain through the years.

"When I was a fellow we had the world's biggest expert on calcium metabolism in premature infants," she recalls. "He'd written thousands of papers. But every time in the nursery I would ask him how to treat a kid—when to treat a kid with hypocalcaemia—he would say, 'We don't know the answer to that.'" Though Cincinnati Children's was known nationally for work on calcium metabolism, some basic treatment questions—*directly affecting children*—remained unanswered.

"Sometimes people answer questions they want to answer as opposed to questions people who are taking care of patients *had* to answer," Kotagal says. "So at that point I said to myself, 'There are a lot of people trying to generate new knowledge. What I'm interested in is how that knowledge gets applied.'"

From Kotagal's perspective, the gap was glaringly obvious. "Why should an organization like this not recognize that we have this knowledge gap? Why would we keep generating this new knowledge without paying attention to whether that knowledge got applied or not, with the same passion as we generated new knowledge?"

As years passed, this question loomed ever larger in her mind. "I was running an intensive care nursery, working harder and harder and I was getting less and less improvement—I had no scientific knowledge of how to *do* [quality improvement]." She found the situation intolerable. She possessed superb clinical skills, but didn't know the first thing about systems or improvement science. She felt she had no choice but to go back to school and learn clinical improvement skills. In 1993, at age forty-five, Uma Kotagal headed to Boston and enrolled in a degree program for a master of science in epidemiology (clinical effectiveness) at the Harvard School of Public Health. Attending classes full-time for two consecutive summers, she learned quantitative skills for clinical research, took courses in epidemiology and biostatistics, and learned how to design and analyze clinical studies. It was demanding work, but she was engaged by it and felt enriched by meeting a variety of faculty and students with whom she discussed a wide array of quality-related issues. It was at Harvard that she met Don Berwick, who taught her a quality improvement course. Uma Kotagal is by nature and inclination a direct person, neither coy nor circuitous in her dealings with people. She told Berwick that she thought his course was boring. Few people told Don Berwick things like that. Typically, in fact, he was a magnetic teacher and speaker, but even on the occasions when he was flat he was cut some slack. Berwick accepted her comment and suggested that perhaps Kotagal was a bit burned out.

"And it was true," she says. But the Harvard experience invigorated her. After earning her degree in 1996, she returned to Cincinnati with renewed determination and newly acquired knowledge. Back at the hospital, she asked the most fundamental question: *What works?* She believed that with common procedures and treatments, she could identify best practices and make sure that particular practice was used every time on every child.

To figure it all out, however, she needed data. She had learned at Harvard that data was essential to quality improvement; that you had to know what aspects of clinical care were going well and what were not before attempting to improve. There were times when care seemed to Kotagal to be more art than science. As a doctor, she understood, of course, that art was an important element of medicine, but there was too little in the way of standard practice—the surest route to consistent quality. And where it was clear what best practices were, she could see a distressing lack of consistency in following them. In the care of preterm newborns, for example, it was established that simple steps increased survival among premature babies, including keeping them warm and administering surfactant to stabilize their lungs. This was not rocket science, but it worked, had been proven to work, and one would think it would be the standard procedure every time. But this was a typical example where the best practice was easily ascertained, yet variation in practice had long existed because no one had systematically sought to identify best practice—or at least a better practice.

"So if we know these things produce healthier children, then why don't we have a system in place to make sure we do it every time for every child?" asks Kotagal. "For example, if we knew kids should get surfactant at four hours, why wouldn't they *all* get it at four hours? If we knew kids shouldn't get cold, why would they get cold anyway? It became really unbearable to know that there was this gap. Kids were getting hurt."

Her response was to start a clinical effectiveness program to see which treatments and procedures were effective and which were ineffective, wasteful, or even potentially harmful. But good data was scarce in health care at the time and she had little choice but to wade through billing records to try to detect patterns of care. It was slow, tedious work, but it was the only data available. She was busy analyzing this jumble of numbers when she was asked to help solve a problem. As the winter of 1995 approached, the hospital anticipated, based on past history, that children with bronchialitis would be admitted in large numbers. They would be treated with chest physiotherapy and nebulizers, increasing demand for the services of respiratory therapists. The expectation, again based on past experience, was that demand would overwhelm supply leaving the ICU short of respiratory therapists.

In tackling the problem, Kotagal started by closely examining the effectiveness of the standard treatment—chest physiotherapy and nebulizers. She wondered about its clinical origin. Was it a proven best practice or a habit passed down through the years? She assembled a small medical team to review the treatment method. In weeks, the team made an important discovery: "Not only were these therapies not effective, but they could be dangerous," she says. "For children with bronchialitis, the primary thing you needed to do was hydrate them and keep them well oxygenated. All this other stuff didn't work." That winter, the hospital through its clinics and physician practices put in place the simple new approach—keeping kids hydrated and oxygenated. The result: Many fewer kids required hospitalization, and the ones who did were in for shorter stays. By applying evidence, Kotagal had succeeded in reducing significant wasteful spending on what were clearly inappropriate hospital admissions. Fueled by success, she created teams and developed treatment guidelines for more than two dozen common childhood illnesses. "It turns out that every time we do something based on evidence, the cost goes down because there's so much waste in the system," she says. "By focusing on quality, we can achieve cost reduction." This was also the case with surgical site infections, where Cincinnati Children's applied the Institute for Healthcare Improvement (IHI) "bundle," a series of specific best-practice steps that had been proven to be the best available evidence-based care. IHI had worked with clinicians throughout the country to develop bundles—processes designed to provide the highest possible quality of care—for a variety of particular treatments, including sepsis, central lines, and ventilators. At Cincinnati Children's, when the IHI bundles were used, site infections were significantly reduced thus reducing the cost of a hospital stay. Kotagal says that "doing the right thing—applying evidence"— saves money. She quickly adds that "not doing things not indicated, as was the case with premature babies, also saves money while increasing the likelihood of positive outcomes."

Sometimes in those early years, Kotagal felt as though she was on her own, that the hospital leadership didn't really understand what she was doing. But that all changed in 1996 and 1997 when a new leadership team took over: Jim Anderson as CEO and Lee Carter as chairman of the board.

It would be difficult to find a CEO and chairman more committed to the quality cause than Anderson and Carter. Unlike most hospital CEOs, Anderson had no health care management or clinical experience before he took the job (though he had been chairman of the Cincinnati Children's Board and was thus intimately familiar with the institution). He had been a practicing attorney as well as president of U.S. operations at Xomox Corporation, a large manufacturer of specialty process controls. As a corporate CEO he possessed a keen understanding of industrial quality improvement techniques and the cultural commitment required for quality.

The sine qua non of quality improvement in health care is leadership. Without the right leadership, quality improvement efforts are, for all practical purposes, doomed. Yet with the right leadership—strong, directed, committed—anything is possible. Anderson, Carter, and Kotagal are well-suited for their roles, but the glue that binds them is a passionate belief and sustained commitment to quality improvement every day for every patient.

"Jim came from industry and he recognized the important quality improvement stuff," says Kotagal. "And he was appalled at the state of healthcare." He liked what Kotagal was doing, and he shifted her within the organization so that she reported directly to him. "Jim wanted standardized results. He saw that in health care we have great products but we don't deliver it every time to every person."

Board chairman Lee Carter is similarly patient-focused (as opposed to focused on finances, a common preoccupation of hospital board members). He also plays a critical role as the avuncular figure, a bit older, more seasoned in the ways of the world, and he balances the relentless drive of Anderson and Kotagal.

"It was clear that people who worked here felt research was more highly valued than patient care," recalls Carter. "We had a research committee on the board and I wanted to add a patient care committee right away." It was not long before Carter got the patient care committee he wanted and it studied "what we were doing well and not doing well."

At meetings of the Cincinnati Children's Hospital board of trustees, the enduring tradition was that the chaplain would begin with a heartwarming story about a child who had faced terrible odds and nearly stared death in the face, only to be saved by the miraculous intervention of Cincinnati Children's clinicians. Jim Anderson, as a member and chairman of the board, heard many of these stories, and they were indeed remarkable. Such stories gave board members a powerful surge of emotion and pride in their association with such an institution.

"We felt good," Anderson recalls. "We never talked about deaths or serious safety events—never anything negative clinically." That changed, of course, when Anderson took over as CEO and Carter as board chairman and they climbed aboard the Uma Kotagal quality improvement express.

"The whole role of the board is to *pay attention*," says Lee Carter. "It's amazing the impact it has when board members go to meetings in the hospital. We're all united from frontline nurse to chairman of the board—we all have the same goal."

As Carter walks through the hallways of the hospital, he greets various employees—nurses, nurses' aides, physicians—by name. He exudes a sense of appreciation for their efforts. Carter's devotion to Cincinnati Children's, like his enthusiasm for the quality journey, is boundless. Around 2005 he was struggling with the idea of defining the hospital's quality mission as precisely as he could. The core of the idea he was wrestling with was that complete transparency reveals that "you are not the best at everything and can always improve." One night he awoke around 3:00 A.M. and the definition came to him: *"We will be the best at getting better."* It precisely defined the Cincinnati Children's aspiration to improve every day "until we are the best and then we will remain the best because we will be the best at getting better."

They were open to change and improvement, eager for new ideas, and one presented itself at Lee Carter's second meeting as board chair when a doctor handed him a brochure and said, "Lee, we need to do more of this." The brochure described an upcoming conference in California about patient- and family-centered care. Carter had never heard of family-centered care, but after speaking with Anderson and Kotagal, he decided that the conference was worth attending. Anderson didn't dispatch a group and direct them to report back. He went himself—along with Carter and several doctors and nurses. At the conference, run by the Institute for Family-Centered Care, they learned from the organization's leader—the dynamic Bev Johnson—that patient- and family-centered health care involves "partnerships among health care patients, families, and providers." It means sharing information so that parents are fully informed. It means that clinicians listen carefully to the personal and cultural preferences for care.

Early on, Kotagal reached out to her old instructor, Don Berwick, who had made several visits to the hospital. On one occasion, he told them they were not tapping the abundance of information available from families. The conference message echoed that sentiment. Elements of family-centered care included respect and dignity; it called for clinicians to share complete information with families on a timely basis, thus enabling families to help make well-informed decisions about care. Believing that families should have immediate access to test results, the hospital created a secure Web portal where families could acquire information—including test results—as soon as it was posted (families and clinicians would receive the same information at precisely the same time). This was more efficient in that it eliminated the middle-man step in which a doctor or nurse would review the results and then call the family to relay the information.

"When we went to the conference it was so clear this was the right thing to do," says Carter. "It was just common sense that we should do this—every other industry listens to its customers–why don't we? We were immersed in stories about how to connect with families and patients—about how to take advantage of their knowledge—especially in the pediatric world where the care giver is the family. And it was clearly not what we were doing."

Before the group attended the conference, the approach to rounds had pointedly excluded parents, who would routinely be asked to leave the child's room while the clinical team conducted its examination. With family-centered rounds, there was a much more intimate and open communication with families. Clinicians on these rounds state clearly what has to happen for the child to be ready to go home, for example. The prerequisites for release are written in plain language on a white board on the room's wall. Clinicians ask patients and family members questions designed to help them understand what is on the family's mind: *How do you feel about this plan? Are you comfortable with it? Do we all agree on this? Are you confident about this? Do you feel okay about it?*

"Now during rounds we say to parents, 'Would you please stay so we can talk and we want to take advantage of your knowledge of your child.' We don't know little five-year-old Ralphie, but Mom knows little Ralphie. We started to use the asset of the parents' knowledge. It's a hugely different approach," says Carter. "Hugely different. Family-centered care acknowledges that families are experts in their children's care."

Jim Anderson wanted to push ahead much further. He needed to place the organization under a microscope and thoroughly scrutinize every aspect of it. He initiated a strategic planning process in which doctors, nurses, administrators, pharmacists, housekeeping staff—everyone who played a role in the hospital—were asked to assess the hospital's strengths, weaknesses, and overall performance. The process, designed to identify goals for the years ahead, commenced in late 1999 with a series of meetings.

At the time, the Cincinnati Children's Hospital self-image was, and had been for many years, one of excellence. There had long been a general conceit among its physician leaders that they were affiliated with one of the finest research facilities in the country—perhaps the world (this general attitude was not at all uncommon in health care: the firm and unsubstantiated belief that *we are among the best*). But at Cincinnati Children's, the self-image was about to be jarred, and not by sniping outsiders but by some of the most prestigious people within the organization. At one of the planning meetings, a surgeon named Robin Cotton, an internationally known pediatric ENT specialist, essentially told the hospital leadership that at Cincinnati Children's *we do not get the high quality outcomes we should. We've got great clinicians but a really bad system.*

Lee Carter had known Robin forever; he could not believe that one of the most respected doctors within the place was saying they were doing a lousy job. Carter turned to Jim Anderson and said, "*Whooaa.*"

The dam then broke. One nurse said the hospital made patients wait way too long. Another said they didn't do a good enough job at pain management. It was shocking, yes, but Jim Anderson immediately saw the outpouring of concern for what it was: an opportunity. Says Anderson: "To have someone from the medical side say basically we need industrial quality was a thrill for me because I understood it—I had lived it. I had seen how clumsily we did things and it was a great relief to me when he said this."

Cotton's remark propelled the strategic planning process in a powerful direction. It gave people throughout the organization the permission and courage to speak candidly—*precisely* what Anderson wanted.

"We will dramatically transform the way we deliver health care at Cincinnati Children's," read the first line of the Cincinnati Children's strategic plan. The words echoed the *Chasm* report.

The plan's language evokes *Chasm* as well—talk of family focus, communication skills, patient safety, minimizing individual blame, redesigning processes for care and access—quality, safety, and effectiveness. A surge of energy and ideas rose within the hospital along with a sense of excitement that so much could be accomplished, and all of that was about to multiply five-fold.

While Kotagal and her team were working on improvement, Don Berwick and his colleagues at IHI had been collaborating with the country's major health care foundation on a dynamic new program. The combination of IHI, which had become *the* health care quality improvement organization, and the Robert Wood Johnson Foundation, the nation's largest philanthropy devoted exclusively to health care, was formidable. The two organizations created a program called Pursuing Perfection; its framework was drawn from the *Chasm* report in which Berwick had played such a pivotal role. Pursuing Perfection goals were drawn directly from *Chasm*'s six aims for improvement: safety, effectiveness, patient-centeredness, timeliness, efficiency, and equity. The RWJ Foundation committed in excess of $20 million to the project. Said Berwick: "The goal of this initiative is to make it possible for patients to be measurably safer, healthier, functioning at higher levels, waiting less time for care and feeling more respected by the health care system."

Just two months after the strategic plan was in place, word of the Pursuing Perfection competition reached Cincinnati Children's. When Uma Kotagal told Jim Anderson about it, his response was: "You mean people will pay us to do what we've committed to do anyway?" Anderson and Kotagal studied the parameters of the program and thought it was a perfect fit for what they were trying to accomplish. Anderson told Kotagal: "We need to win this grant."

But the competition was ferocious. Word soon came that more than 200 hospitals had applied, that 12 would be chosen for a brief phase I program, and just 7 would make the final cut. The application required hospitals to identify two clinical areas they sought to improve and to outline how they intended to go about it. Kotagal was in charge of putting the application together, though the timing for her was unfortunate. She was leaving for a long-planned trip to India and it could not be put off. Before departing, she put together a core team of two doctors, Maria Britto and Keith Mandel, and a nurse, Gerry Pandzik. Leaders of the pulmonary division agreed to join in and help seek the grant (they wanted to focus on cystic fibrosis), but Kotagal had difficulty in getting any other clinical areas interested in the project.

"We went to a number of different people who said, 'No, we don't know what you're talking about'—who didn't understand what the project was about. Others thought it would just be too much extra work and wanted no part of it."

Kotagal finally settled on a bronchiolitis project intended to "establish a system for acute care delivery that is family-centered and evidence-based." The cystic fibrosis (CF) project aimed to work with CF patients and families to design and implement "a comprehensive delivery system for children and adolescents." With Kotagal writing portions of the grant proposal from India and the rest of her team working back in Cincinnati, they succeeded in putting together what they thought was a fairly impressive proposal. A few months later, they were thrilled to learn that they had been selected for a site visit.

Kotagal and Anderson learned in advance that the site visit would include Maureen Bisognano, the IHI chief operating officer, and Robert Brook, MD, head of the health care division at RAND. Bisognano is the consummate professional: smart, tough-minded, but warm and affable. Brook, on the other hand, "tends to get a little gruff."

Kotagal worked hard to prepare with the group engaging in formal rehearsals under the guidance of a presentation consultant. Their preparation indicated how high the stakes were for Cincinnati Children's. There was the $2 million grant money, which could pay for a lot of quality improvement, but much more than that there was the promise of working with some of the leading quality experts in the world through IHI. There would also be an opportunity to learn from other health care organizations carefully chosen by IHI as seriously committed to the quality journey.

On the day of the visit, things got ugly fast. Lee Carter had barely begun his well-rehearsed introduction when Brook, in a none-too-pleasant tone, challenged him. As Kotagal recalls, "Lee said welcome and started it off and Bob said something like, 'So, what do *you* know about the safety record for this hospital?' And Lee probably knew more than most chairmen of the board, but Bob wouldn't stop. He just grilled Lee, and he really grilled Jim, and he and Jim had this little tension where Jim said, 'I'm going to say what I'm going to say.'"

Brook sat there picking up his folder and then dropping it in a combination of what appeared frustration and disgust. "He was like a little kid who visibly wanted you to know he was bored," says Kotagal.

It was clear the meeting was verging on disaster, and then it got worse. Brook looked around the room at the Cincinnati Children's team and said, as Kotagal recalls, "'Okay, so you're all here and the evidence is pretty clear that writing [prescription] orders causes harm, so why don't you issue an edict today . . . that all orders will be typed.' Then somebody said something like, 'We don't have those errors,' which of course was an absolutely ridiculous thing to say."

At that point, Kotagal, who had sat steaming silently throughout, decided to speak up. "I finally said, 'You know you can always ask these questions and trap people in the answers, but I'm hoping that's not what you're here to do—that this is not a pimping kind of academic exercise, because that's what it feels like, and I hope what you're here to know is whether we are of the passion and commitment to do this. And if we had the answers why would you be here?'"

Kotagal had thought Brook rude, but she understood that he had, in a sense, earned the right to be ornery. He was, after all, one of the giants of the quality improvement world, one of the pioneers, and his patience had worn perilously thin through the years—through the decades, in fact. He did not like seeing patients hurt and he did not like seeing patients go without the care they needed.

"He is a brilliant guy, a classic academic," says Kotagal. . . . "You could see he only had three hours and he had to figure out if this was going to work or not work. And basically I think he concluded we had the passion and interest and commitment even though we didn't have a clue."

The call from Don Berwick and Maureen Bisognano at IHI came first thing in the morning. Anticipating word, Kotagal had gathered the team together around a speaker phone. She looked around at these very serious, unflappable professionals—Jim Anderson, Maria Britto, Keith Mandel, and others—and could see the tension. And then the word came: They had won! The usually unflappable professionals cheered, hugged, and high-fived one another like school kids. They had been selected for several reasons. Berwick and Bisognano had been impressed by the steely certainty of their commitment and their passion for the work. But the clincher was the Cincinnati Children's leadership. When Maureen Bisognano and Bob Brook had gone in for the site visit, there sat the chairman of the board and CEO. That certainly didn't happen everywhere else. And Bisognano did not have to spend long with Dr. Kotagal before knowing that she was a change agent.

In the first phase of the project, September 2001 to March 2002, they would receive a grant of $50,000 to plan the improvement projects. Their excitement was tempered by the knowledge that although twelve organizations had been selected for phase I, only seven would move on to the far more robust phase II. Within

Kotagal's team, a competitive instinct was aroused; its members wanted to perform well enough on phase I to win selection to phase II, a major two-year project (April 2002 through March 2004). Those selected would each receive nearly $2 million in funding to underwrite some of the improvement efforts. Berwick and his IHI colleagues, along with Robert Wood Johnson Foundation, had set a goal as ambitious as anything being done in health care quality improvement anywhere in the country—perhaps the world. Those receiving grants were expected to "implement broad and comprehensive quality improvement plans throughout their organizations . . . leading to organizational transformation."

"The first thing it gave us was legitimacy," recalls Kotagal. "For an academic organization, that's important. I could use the grant as a mechanism to fund faculty. I had a small core team, Maria Britto, Keith Mandel, Jerry Kaminski, Gerry Pandzik, Bill Kent, and myself. We met every week for two hours and that was the design team. Everybody on that team worked hundreds of hours, read stuff, each weekend we'd read two to three books to know what's out there."

Jim Anderson saw Pursuing Perfection "as the engine that drives the transformational change that is necessary for us to become the leader in improving child health." It became, perhaps more than anything else, an intensive learning experience. Cincinnati Children's established two pilot projects for pursuing perfect health care: children with an acute condition (bronchiolitis), and children with a chronic condition (cystic fibrosis). But among the most important lessons Kotagal and her team learned had nothing to do with either CF or bronchiolitis. "We learned a lot about how difficult it was to do this in healthcare and how difficult it was to do it in an academic organization where research was the currency and fixing systems was viewed as somewhat sloppy and fuzzy," she says. "We knew at that point in time that we had to create a respect for the science of improvement for it to survive in the organization."

The IHI help was key for Kotagal. "We were overwhelmed by the immense nature of the project," she recalls. Berwick and IHI connected Kotagal with Tom Nolan, a PhD statistician and expert in quality improvement. Nolan was close to Berwick and Maureen Bisognano and had played a pivotal role in their thinking about the mission of IHI. Nolan had a long history of work in industry, but had been drawn into health care and IHI. Kotagal characterizes Nolan as "hugely important" in the organization's improvement journey by helping to apply solid science and measurement to their efforts. With Nolan's statistical expertise, they were measuring outcomes instead of guessing. Says Kotagal: "If I have a voice whispering in my head, it's Tom's voice. I've learned more from Tom than I have from anybody. From Don, I've learned about the passion and the openness and the deep commitment. From Tom, I've learned a cool-headed kind of methods approach."

IHI also brought Kotagal and her colleagues together with other national experts who were essential in guiding them forward. From Dartmouth came Paul Batalden's colleague Gene Nelson to advise on measurement. From RAND came, of all people, the legendary Bob Brook on, as Kotagal put it, "what was possible to think about."

The triumvirate of Anderson, Carter, and Kotagal was critical to change, says Nolan. With Jim Anderson as CEO and his industrial experience, "he wasn't bound by the status quo as maybe some CEOs who had spent their whole careers in health care might have been." He adds, "They were very curious—especially Uma—about how modern methods of improvement could be applied in an academic medical center. It was much like where Don and Paul Batalden were fifteen years earlier—solid citizens in health care but curious about new methods."

An essential part of the program involved participants convening for regular meetings to exchange ideas and discuss what they were learning. Often it wasn't the big items but small ideas for improvement that could apply to almost any hospital. During the meetings, Kotagal found herself over and over again hearing about a small step involving patient safety or quality and remarking, "Oh, that could work for us."

"Pursuing Perfection helped them a lot," observes Tom Nolan. "They're good learners. They picked the best and went with it."

"With *Pursuing Perfection,* Uma was off and running," says Jim Anderson. In taking the reins of improvement work at Cincinnati Children's, Kotagal drove the employees with a passion that alternately inspired, exasperated, and exhausted her troops. She can grow quite impatient when results are not forthcoming and she is "constantly driving, driving, driving people to a higher level," says Dr. Keith Mandel. Jim Anderson agrees: "She won't lower standards. She will not let people off the hook." In her view, he says, "there is no excuse to not provide better care to kids." As tough as she is on people, she is ultimately more inspirational than anything. Lee Carter describes her as "our Berwick."

And she saw clearly during the Pursuing Perfection experience that transforming the way care was delivered would require intensive training and education for the staff. In fact, Pursuing Perfection anticipated the need for such training. One of the finest quality improvement courses anywhere in the country had been taught for many years at Intermountain Health Care in Salt Lake City by Brent James, MD, who made available his classes to Pursuing Perfection participants at a discounted rate. Kotagal had met James through Don Berwick when she had taken James's class at the Harvard School of Public Health.

"One of the things you learn in Brent's class is that you have to learn by doing," Kotagal says. "We had to do a project. We were exposed to the fundamental knowledge of how you improve systems."

Kotagal identified seven people from Cincinnati Children's she wanted to take to Salt Lake. Obvious choices included Maria Britto, chief of staff Mike Farrell, and others, all of whom had played a significant role in putting together the Pursuing Perfection application. She also included Susie Allen, the physician in charge of nursing development and co-leader of the diabetes team.

But Kotagal also wanted to include Fred Ryckman, MD, which would not be easy. Dr. Ryckman was renowned at Cincinnati Children's—and beyond—for the surgical transplant program he had created there. Ryckman was one of the most productive, and profitable, surgeons at the hospital and the idea of taking him to the Brent James classes—a commitment of two full weeks per month for three months—seemed madness. It was certainly counter to anything that would even have been contemplated in the past or at just about any other hospital in the country.

"I started the transplant lab and it was my life for fifteen years," Ryckman says. "I was working with my head down focused only on the job of transplanting organs into very sick children, many of them tiny infants"—some as small as five pounds.

Although it seemed on the surface to make no sense to take Ryckman out of his role to engage in quality improvement education, Kotagal had a method to her madness. She intentionally recruited some of the highest profile and most respected people within the organization, reasoning that if she could convert these people to the quality movement it would be taken much more seriously by the rest of the employees. It was, of course, a high-risk strategy. Ryckman was, like Kotagal, a very direct person. If, for example, he should return from Salt Lake City and pronounce the course a waste of time, Kotagal's quality work might be doomed right then and there. Fortunately, he had the opposite reaction. "When we went to Salt Lake to Brent James's class I walked into it totally blind," says Ryckman. During the course, guest lecturers taught various segments. After one guest speaker had addressed the class, Ryckman turned to Kotagal and said: "Wow, that guy is really smart—who is he?"

"He's the head of IHI," Kotagal replied. "His name is Don Berwick."

For Ryckman, it was a transforming experience:

I had spent my whole career doing what I needed to do *today* to try and save this kid's life. I was used to devoting eighteen hours for one person. Remove the liver in a donor in two or three hours, take it to the sickest kid, put in the new liver (nine or ten hours of surgery just a few years ago; now down to just three to four hours). I had worked on single individual patients. I remember sitting there in Salt Lake City and thinking if I could work on solving some of these quality problems you're talking about *hundreds* of patients. The question was how can we do systems management and impact hundreds, *thousands* of patients?

Ryckman returned to Cincinnati eager to apply what he had learned. At Kotagal's suggestion, Ryckman immediately began working on surgical site infections. He did not initially think it was a problem in his own area: "We thought we were doing it right in my area 95 percent of the time." But measurement soon revealed (and they had never measured this before) that it was closer to 65 or 70 percent of the time. In a way, this gave him greater credibility when he went to other departments to push improvement. Other surgeons would tell him they were positive their areas were doing surgical sites correctly 90-plus percent of the time.

"That's what I thought," he would tell them. And the fact that it was Ryckman, a man so widely admired and respected within the organization, caused other doctors to take it seriously. Invariably, in department after department, measurement would reveal a surgical site infection rate far above what the clinicians in that area had thought. Ryckman adopted the IHI surgical site bundle and began applying it in his own department while persuading others to do the same. But this was not easy because the IHI bundle involved a significant amount of effort to change work flows.

"For this to work you had to be 99 percent on every one of the sixteen steps in the IHI bundle every single day with every single patient," says Ryckman.

Then, Kotagal threw a new and, to Ryckman, most unwelcome wrinkle into the work. At the suggestion of Tom Nolan, she wanted Ryckman to produce measurement of surgical site infections every day. Ryckman bristled; this was overdoing it, pushing too hard too fast. But Kotagal would not yield. Any antibiotic failures—increasing the risk of infections—had to be reported daily. This would mean Ryckman going to each surgical group and confronting them for the information—every day.

"Surgeons aren't used to people telling us what to do," says Ryckman with a smile. "A surgeon is a little bit of a loner—to have somebody come to you in the last week and say five times 'this was not done right—how come?' That's not the type of encounters surgeons are used to."

But it was soon clear to Ryckman why Kotagal had insisted on daily measurement. "We could see the failures right away," he says. "Daily data was a key driver. We knew *immediately* when there was a problem."

On top of it all, Kotagal wanted Ryckman to set a goal. He looked at the national data and found that Class 2 surgeries—which included most operations—had an infection rate of between 4 and 5 (out of every hundred surgeries). Cincinnati Children's was much better: between 1.5 and 2. When Kotagal asked what Ryckman thought his target rate should be, he suggested below 2. She dismissed that out of hand.

"What about 0.5?" she asked.

"Much too low," he objected.

She pushed.

He pushed back.

She pushed harder. Ryckman had known Uma Kotagal for twenty years, ever since they had trained together in pediatrics, and he knew she would not back off. And even though he thought "this was the most absurd thing I've ever heard of in my life, I agreed to do it if it would get me a moment of peace."

And so it was settled: The official goal was 0.5 infections per hundred. As the work proceeded, Ryckman found himself checking the daily results and watching, over time, as the overall rate began to decline and move steadily lower. After several months, some of the results were in. The national rate for Class 2 surgery was from 4 to 5, and Cincinnati was between 1.5 and 2; but Ryckman's new results, after the IHI bundle had been applied, were 0.4.

Point four, he thought when he saw it. Amazing.

Ryckman laughs heartily at the recollection of his belief that 0.5 was impossible; he is now convinced that with continued diligence, it might be possible to get as low as 0.2. Ryckman's success stemmed from his use of the basic IHI bundle—intended for adult patients—which he modified to apply in pediatrics. Once Ryckman identified the best practice derived from the IHI prescription, the key was to make it standard work: Apply it every time every day for every patient. It was reminiscent of the work Rick Shannon had done at Allegheny—identify the best practice and apply it every time.

Five years before Ryckman, Kotagal and the others took the Brent James class—before applying the IHI bundle—Ryckman says that clinicians simply would not have believed that lowering the infection rate was even possible. Back then, clinicians would have reacted with a shrug: "Kids get infections; there are a lot of sick kids here. It happens." This, too, was reminiscent of Rick Shannon's experience and echoed his theory about the myth of inevitability, the notion that not much can be done to prevent these infections; that they are inevitable complications in the practice of medicine.

The early projects, perhaps particularly Ryckman's leadership ⟨ the successful surgical site infection issue, generated significant buzz throughout the hospital. People began to get excited about tackling a variety of improvement projects.

Along the way, there were some rocky times. In 2003 and 2004, the organization was subjected to some painful scrutiny—first in the form of PBS series "Remaking American Medicine," which described some of the care at the hospital, and the second in the form of an article in the *New Yorker* magazine focused on cystic fibrosis care at the hospital. Jim Anderson and Lee Carter distinctly recall the moment in the video that stung them both so deeply. A Cincinnati Children's nurse said she had a child with CF and that she had been bringing her child to the hospital for treatment. And she said something that Jim Anderson, Lee Carter, and Uma Kotagal will never forget: "I never bring her in that they don't make a mistake." Anderson shakes his head at the recollection and takes a deep breath. "It leaves me speechless," he says softly. Lee Carter's reaction is the same: "It was like getting kicked in the stomach," he says.

The *New Yorker* article, by Atul Gawande, a Boston surgeon on the magazine staff, was not a dissimilar experience. In the past when Cincinnati Children's was mentioned in the national press, the coverage had typically been positive—consistently ranking near the top of the annual *US News* ratings, for example. And for generations the hospital had held the belief that it was among the finest pediatric institutions in the country—in the world, really.

"The Bell Curve: What Happens When Patients Find Out How Good Their Doctors Really Are?" appeared in the December 6, 2004, issue and ran to a length of nearly 8,000 words, ten times the length of an average newspaper column. In the article, Gawande wrote of a family—the Pages—and their reaction to learning their daughter had cystic fibrosis. "The one overwhelming thought in the minds of Honor and Don Page was: We need to get to Children's." Gawande notes that not only was Cincinnati Children's generally considered one of the "most respected pediatric hospitals in the country," but it was also the home of a pediatrician who had written "the chapter on cystic fibrosis in the *Nelson Textbook of Pediatrics*—the bible of the specialty." The assumption by the Pages was, of course, that Cincinnati Children's was among the leaders in the treatment of cystic fibrosis. Gawande notes that, although the Cincinnati Children's clinicians gave the Pages much information, they held something back:

> The one thing that the clinicians failed to tell them, however, was that Cincinnati Children's was not, as the Pages supposed, among the country's best centers for children with cystic fibrosis. According to data from that year, it was, at best, an average program. . . . By some measures, Cincinnati was well below average. The best predictor of a CF patient's life expectancy is his or her lung function. At Cincinnati, lung function for patients under the age of twelve . . . was in the bottom 25 percent of the country's CF patients. And the doctors there knew it.

In the late winter of 2001, writes Gawande, "the Pages and twenty other families were invited by their doctors at Cincinnati Children's to a meeting about the CF program there." The purpose of the meeting was for doctors to disclose to parents the results of Cincinnati Children's clinical outcomes on CF. This included revealing where Cincinnati Children's ranked compared with other CF programs throughout the country. It was one of the hardest things any of the clinicians had ever had to do—stand up in front of the families with whom they had grown so close and reveal the embarrassing results of their program. But given the improvement journey Cincinnati Children's had embarked upon, there was no other choice. Lee Carter wholeheartedly supported the decision to disclose the information.

"We're honest and we're open," he says. "People understand if you make a mistake; they don't understand if you cover it up. Our whole journey is driven by two factors—family-centered care and transparency."

Parents were alarmed by the statistics, but, perhaps surprisingly, none of the families left the Cincinnati Children's program. Why? Primarily familiarity and trust. Given the amount of care CF requires, families and clinicians were in almost constant contact. Week in and week out for years families had seen how devoted these doctors, nurses, technicians, and others were to their sick children. When the Cincinnati Children's team said they were going to change—promised to become among the best in the country—the parents believed them.

Perhaps there was also another reason. A key component of the improvement process would involve parents of children suffering from CF. Anderson, Carter, and Kotagal, along with other clinicians at the hospital, were convinced that the voice of parents was essential not just occasionally but in an official and sustained way. The result was that parents were included as full participating members of every CF team. This was not an easy decision. Including parents on working groups within pediatric hospitals ranged from rare to unheard of. The attitude in many places was that parents don't really know much, could slow things down, and could actually impede the process of improving care. But at Cincinnati Children's the inherent value of parents—with their enormous stores of knowledge about their children and the diseases they faced—was considered a precious asset.

Kotagal considers it an historic moment for the organization because it was the first time patients were included in such a robust way; and, "although we have modified how we have patients help us in the design, we no longer have any doubts about having them at the table."

Now came the hard part: figuring out how to get better, *much* better, at treating CF patients. This was particularly difficult since Cincinnati

Children's genuinely believed they had been doing everything right. Wrote Gawande: "Not only had the center followed national guidelines for CF; two of its physicians had helped write them."

To learn, the Cincinnati Children's teams wanted to study the approaches of the top-ranked CF centers in the country. But when they asked for the names of those institutions, the Cystic Fibrosis Foundation, keeper of the statistics, refused to disclose the information. Of the 117 CF centers across the country, the Cincinnati Children's team had no idea which were the best. Until, that is, Don Berwick learned that the foundation had refused to disclose the information to them. As Gawande wrote in the *New Yorker:*

> In early 2002, Don Berwick visited the Cincinnati program. He was impressed by its seriousness, and by the intense involvement of the families, but he was incredulous when he learned that the committee couldn't get the names of the top programs from the foundation. He called the foundation's executive vice-president for medical affairs, Preston Campbell. "I was probably a bit self-righteous," Berwick says. "I said, 'How could you do this?' And he said . . . [t]he reason they have done so for forty years is that they have trusted that it would be kept confidential. Once the centers lost that faith, they might no longer report solid, honest information tracking how different treatments are working, how many patients there are, and how well they do.

Soon after Berwick's call, the foundation disclosed to the Cincinnati Children's team the names of the top five CF performers in the country. They began the arduous work of studying the top centers and applying key lessons back in Cincinnati.

Since the disclosure of the results in 2001, Cincinnati Children's results on CF have improved significantly. In the very first year of the improvement project, the organization's rank went from one hundredth in the country to fiftieth. They did it by learning from the University of Minnesota, which scored near the top in the foundation's rankings. A Cincinnati Children's team—including a physician, nurse, nutritionist, and parent—went to learn from the people in Minnesota and adopted their methods.

An essential aspect of quality is managing the care not just of individuals but of populations, just as Cincinnati Children's is doing with its model asthma program. One of Kotagal's protégés, Keith Mandel, who played a key role in winning the Pursuing Perfection grant, runs Tri State Child Health Services, a pediatric Physician-Hospital Organization (PHO) affiliated with Cincinnati Children's. Mandel and his team work on a variety of quality improvement projects with a focus on coordination among primary care physicians, community specialists, and specialty teams at Cincinnati Children's. Mandel began the project in October 2003, and it now includes forty-four community-based primary care practices, 165 pediatricians, and 15,000 children with asthma. Part of the effort involves a pay-for-performance program with a local insurer aimed at rewarding improvement for the asthma population. The program is designed to reward physician groups (rather than individual doctors) for effective management of their collective asthma patients, not merely for doing procedures. Mandel says measurement has been essential to the success of the program. Primary care practices know precisely where they stand on a variety of measures and a healthy sense of competition has developed among the forty-four practices. Mandel has also enlisted school-based nurses in the program in an attempt to reach all children with asthma.

The foundation of the program is getting physicians to administer evidence-based care to asthma patients to keep them healthy and thus reduce work and school absences, emergency-room visits, and hospital admissions. The project involved assembling an asthma team at each practice—doctor, nurse, and office manager—and collecting

comprehensive data on each patient. Mandel and his colleagues relied on a Web-based asthma registry with an array of process and outcomes measures at the overall network level as well as the physician
practice level, thus allowing comparison between and among various
physician groups. This sort of transparent data fueled competition
among the groups—clearly to the benefit of patients (without such
data, there is no real competition). Another key part of the effort involved a campaign to increase the percentage of asthma patients receiving flu shots. The results of the program have been outstanding
yielding a 50 percent reduction in hospital admissions for pediatric
asthma patients, a 24 percent reduction in school days missed, and a
30 percent reduction in work days missed by parents.

Although the program has been successful thus far, the folks at
Cincinnati Children's believe they can do much better, particularly
with adolescents afflicted with asthma and, more particularly, with
inner-city adolescents with asthma. Maria Britto, MD, a member of
Kotagal's team that prepared the Pursuing Perfection application and
an expert in chronic diseases, is a rising star at Cincinnati Children's
and in many ways reminiscent of Dr. Kotagal. Britto trained in internal medicine and pediatrics and was chief resident of pediatrics at
the University of North Carolina Hospitals, where she earned a master's degree in public health in epidemiology. An indication of her
brilliance was her selection for the prestigious Robert Wood Johnson
Clinical Scholars Program.

In 2007, Britto won approval to build a new entity within the hospital called the Center for Innovation in Chronic Disease Care. Its
mission is to identify and break down barriers preventing adolescents
from following the appropriate clinical path. Britto and colleagues
targeted the toughest asthma population—urban adolescents—many
poor, most African American. Since getting these kids to take their
medicine in a consistent and timely fashion is a huge problem, Britto
is working to teach better self-management skills to them and also

trying to determine what specific steps she can take to keep them out of the emergency room. "We want to provide nearly perfect evidence-based care, make kids confident, and keep them from having activity limitations," she says.

Britto noticed how frequently adolescent patients sent and received text messages. This would happen throughout the exam with some kids, and it struck Britto that she should communicate with the kids in the manner they chose. She and her innovation team set up a program of text-message reminders to adolescents to take their medicine. Kids signing up for the program would receive any number of reminders at various times of the day. Not long thereafter, one of her patients came in for a regularly scheduled appointment and it turned out that he had been using his inhaler twice a day as recommended. Britto was surprised because he had never shown any consistency in the past. "How did you remember to do that?" she asked, and he pulled out his phone: "It's the text messages you send me every day."

Other cases, she is finding, are much harder. She has a patient—a seventeen-year-old boy—who consumes huge quantities of medication and yet winds up in the ER just about every week. Britto was puzzled by the case because the boy's asthma, although problematic, was certainly not as bad as that of many other patients. "We'd see him Tuesday and he'd be in the ER Wednesday," she says.

Britto tried an experiment: She told the boy she would see him any time he wanted. She also asked him a question: What would you like us to do for you that we are not now doing? He asked for a nebulizer, and she gave him one. She set up appointments wherever he wanted, seeing him even though he showed up two and a half hours late for an appointment. At one point, as she was helping him, he seemed to grow alarmed: "Does this mean I'm not getting admitted?" he asked.

His lack of compliance and self-management, it became clear, centered on anxiety. He felt safer and more protected inside the hospital than out. He was comforted by his nearly continuous connection with the medical establishment. Britto connected him to a therapist to help treat his anxiety, but she says the most important lesson was that she had demonstrated to him that Cincinnati Children's would do whatever it took to meet his needs, help him manage his disease, and keep him healthy.

"Eighty percent of the kids don't need that level of help but twenty percent do," says Britto. "It's a small group of patients who have disproportional needs, who use a lot of resources and don't have good outcomes." She aims to get at this population, and at least anecdotally, she has had some success.

This particular boy, after some counseling went from being in the ER twice a week on average to once in five months. Was it worth it to reach out and provide so much time and energy for this patient? No doubt. First, he is on a far better track with his disease, and doing much better at self-management. He is also staying out of the hospital, which means he is staying in school and saving the health care system significant dollars.

With the Center for Innovation in Chronic Disease Care, Britto and her colleagues are providing clinical treatment while they conduct research to determine the best ways to treat these kids. Her hope is that they will come up with approaches that work well in asthma and can be used with asthma patients throughout the country. Beyond that, she aspires to find methods of treatment that can be applied to other chronic diseases as well. As part of her effort to get kids to take their medicine, her team recently added a simple question to the short list each patient is asked at the beginning of a clinical visit: "Is there anything going on in your life that makes it especially difficult to manage your asthma?"

This prompted some interesting, often surprising answers. One fourteen-year-old patient replied: "Yes. I'm in a gang and whenever I think I might get shot my asthma gets worse." It turned out that he had been in the gang since he was not quite twelve years old and wanted out. Britto and her team were able to connect him with a social service agency to help him do just that. She realized that to provide the kind of care these adolescents needed she had to probe more to determine whether underlying issues, if solved, would enable them to control their disease and live a healthier life.

Within an original trial group of a hundred patients, Britto and her team covered three key process measures with 98 percent of the kids (getting the disease characterized; putting kids with persistent disease on medication; and creating an asthma action plan). With clinical measures, however, they have a long way to go. Only fifteen of the hundred kids have their disease completely controlled. Her goal is to reach 60 percent. She believes that "if we do all the self-management stuff right" they can reach the goal. But it is grueling, patient-by-patient work.

In spite of all the work and all the progress, Cincinnati Children's still makes mistakes—too many mistakes. Thus, patient safety has become the hospital's top priority. Asked why, Steve Muething, the physician in charge of the safety project, replies: "Because the fact that we harm a kid every twenty days is difficult to swallow."

An essential element of the hospital's safety effort is transparency. Cincinnati Children's publishes the details of serious safety events on its Web site and displays the number of days since the most recent event—rare among hospitals anywhere. Muething emphasizes the importance of the hospital's leadership in promoting safety and observes that both Jim Anderson and Lee Carter "believe that admitting our weaknesses and facing up to our mistakes is critical to improving." Muething notes that "they personally OK'd the decision" to reveal details of serious safety events publicly, and adds: "I am pretty sure no other hospital in the U.S. is sharing that information daily."

When Kotagal placed Dr. Muething in charge of the safety project, he researched other hospitals around the country, and was captivated by the work at Sentara, a six-hospital system based in Norfolk, Virginia. "The number one item I saw at Sentara was data," he recalls. "They shared a run chart of their last several years of Serious Safety Events. I was struck by two things. First they were willing to share data on an item that almost every other hospital said was absolutely confidential [serious safety events]. Second, they had a plan that explained results to date and how they were moving forward."

As Paul Batalden and Don Berwick had done a couple of decades earlier, Sentara looked to other industries for guidance, drawing upon safety practices from aviation and nuclear power to build a powerful safety culture. Much of it involves common sense, yet applied systematically it has a real impact. The basic Sentara approach is the STAR method—"Stop for a few seconds to concentrate on the particular task; think about the task; act or perform the task; review or double check to ensure that the task was completed correctly." When words sound alike, Sentara staff members are explicit. After saying that a medication requires fourteen milligrams, they will add: "That's one, four, not four, zero." Handoffs during shift changes are crucial moments when a lack of communication can lead to mistakes. Sentara focuses intensively on handoffs breaking down the process into categories of information that make for a successful handoff—called the Five Ps: "The Patient or Project that is handed off, the Plan that is to be implemented, the Purpose of the task, any Problems that can occur and any Precautions that should be taken with the particular patient or project."

When Muething saw the work at Sentara, he picked up the phone and called Kotagal back in Cincinnati. "I think I just saw it," he said. When he returned to Cincinnati, he went to work immediately implementing much of the plan from Sentara.

Muething regularly writes informal dispatches to the Cincinnati Children's community on various safety topics. They are engaging in their simple directness and important as reminders of the ubiquitous perils in hospitals. He emphasizes the importance of a time-out just prior to an invasive procedure when those involved go through an airline-like checklist to make sure everything is exactly right. In one of his safety journals, Muething wrote about a child who was facing a procedure in radiology. In the room were physicians, nurses, and a child life specialist—a young woman at the bottom of the clinical hierarchy. For some reason the time-out had been skipped, and with the procedure about to start, she called a halt—empowered to do so by the Cincinnati Children's safety rules. She said they could not proceed until a full and careful time-out had been completed. As Muething observed: "Rather than assuming that this was a 'doctor thing' or a 'nurse thing,' the child life specialist spoke up and reminded the team that they needed to carry out the time-out to be safe for this child and family."

Perhaps the story here is a cultural one—the empowerment of non-physicians at Cincinnati Children's. Not so many years ago, the notion that anyone but a doctor would flex his muscles in the OR was unthinkable. But quality and safety depend upon the whole team; and although many institutions across the country have not yet realized this, some clearly have. Muething reported on two nurses who,

> in the "old days," worried about safety, especially when they saw others acting in a way that might increase risk to the patient. But they usually didn't say anything. It wasn't because they didn't care. It was because they were nervous, didn't want to cause trouble, felt someone else would speak up, didn't want to get barked at, etc. I think that's the way most of us approached patient safety. I know I did.

But in two cases, these two nurses stepped in and took control in situations in which they felt procedure was not being followed and a patient might be at risk.

As with most change in health care, this sounds easier than it is. Even at a place like Cincinnati Children's, change comes with conflict, tension, and pushback. Muething says there are still people in his hospital who "rush through time-outs in the operating room or . . . get angry at a colleague who points out they forgot to wash their hands or they don't report a safety concern because it's not important."

Muething is relentless, though. He studied the concept of Red Rules in industrial safety—rules that could never be violated under any circumstances. After some reflection, Muething realized that a time-out prior to a surgical procedure should happen 100 percent of the time; that to fail to have a time-out risked harm to the patient that was entirely preventable. Thus he established Cincinnati Children's first Red Rule: time-outs before every invasive procedure.

There are always clinicians, however, resistant to standardization. Some doctors are impatient with such procedures, dismissive of them as a waste of time. Over a series of months, a great majority of surgeons had signed on to the program, but not enough to satisfy Muething. Then there was a serious safety event that could have been prevented by a time-out. And then another. And then a third—and Muething had had enough. In December 2007, Muething—along with Jim Anderson and Uma Kotagal—met with the ten surgical chiefs. Muething, along with Anderson and Kotagal, made it clear that the Red Rule was inviolate and they needed the chiefs to enforce it 100 percent of the time in their areas. This meeting was followed by a mandatory gathering of all 300 surgeons working at Cincinnati Children's in the ten clinical areas. They gathered in the hospital auditorium, where Muething, Anderson, and Kotagal were on the stage. Muething had brought the hospital's attorneys. He explained that there would be zero tolerance for any surgeon who violated the policy; that they were required to agree to the policy and to abide by it; that if they chose not to agree, they were free to leave the staff. And every surgeon—then and there in the auditorium—was required to sign a statement that they would agree to a time-out before every procedure.

Cincinnati Children's has advanced to the point where Kotagal is now focused on learning "how to do improvement." She adds, "We don't want to learn anymore about the content, we want to learn *how* you do this." Tom Nolan and his colleague Lloyd Provost guide Kotagal and her team as they think about, as Kotagal puts it, "the next steps, and the next steps, and the next steps."

She has developed a quality improvement course internally at Cincinnati Children's modeled on Brent James's class. No longer does she feel the necessity to send new quality recruits to Salt Lake City. "We teach about thirty people at a time," she says. "We didn't want to start the class until we had enough stories to tell. One of the things about Brent's course was the stories . . . so you could hear about this person and what project they did, and how they struggled and what results they got, and that was as important as learning the method."

Anderson, Carter, and Kotagal all believe they have made a powerful business case for quality improvement. Cincinnati Children's has grown financially 16 percent a year for ten years, "and we could not have done it without quality improvement." In 2006, Cincinnati Children's was awarded the American Hospital Association-McKesson Quest for Quality Prize. Symbolically, the prize was a recognition for all the work they have done through the years—a nice bit of recognition for the long quality journey young Dr. Kotagal started when she was an impatient fellow in neonatology thirty years ago. The language of the award sums up the Cincinnati Children's story very nicely: "Cincinnati Children's . . . has completely engrained quality improvement and excellence and all six of the Institute of Medicine's quality aims into its institutional culture . . . [and] has made major strides in patient-centeredness, uses evidence-based guidelines, strives to address racial disparities in their community and uses data very effectively."

Hospitals throughout the country and the world can learn a great deal from Cincinnati Children's. A week never passes during which they do not host visitors from other medical centers hoping to learn from them.

The question for so many of these organizations is this: What is the formula for success in quality improvement? There are small moments when a clinician discovers a process or procedure—nothing dramatic, but something meaningful—something that works better than what was done before; something that in some small way makes life better for the patient. The journey is marked by discovery and disappointment and perseverance in the face of that disappointment. It is marked by moments of drama, key turning points without which the process might go awry. It is marked by years and years of work. Most of all—more important than anything else—it is marked by leadership, persistence, and a passion to improve.

7

Virginia Mason Medical Center and the Toyota Production System

"The patient is God."

Gary Kaplan, MD, had specialized in internal medicine at Virginia Mason Medical Center (VMMC) in Seattle ever since arriving there as a resident in 1978. He was widely respected as a fine clinician and admired for his ability to work cooperatively with a variety of groups and individuals. In 2000, when Kaplan was forty-eight years old, his reputation for teamwork, effectiveness, and integrity, seasoned with a fair bit of charisma, helped elevate him to chairman and CEO, just the seventh in the eighty-year history of Virginia Mason. When Kaplan took over, Virginia Mason was a not-for-profit regional health care system employing nearly 500 physicians working in a 336-bed acute care hospital; it also included numerous clinics throughout the Puget Sound area. The center was also coming off two down financial years, having lost a lot of money in 1998 and 1999. "There was a sense of crisis," says Kaplan.

Early on, Kaplan wanted an independent, clear-eyed assessment of precisely where the company stood. Along with the board of directors, he attended a retreat where consultants from Kaufman Hall, a health care consulting firm, outlined the type of financial performance needed for medical centers to prosper.

"It was a rude awakening," recalls Kaplan. "We saw the kinds of economic ratios that were required to sustain ourselves and invest in our facilities and we were falling short."

Soon after the retreat, Kaplan addressed a gathering of the Virginia Mason professional staff as bluntly as he could: "We change," he said, "or we die." There was no alternative, he said, but to change the way VMMC was doing business. Greater financial discipline was essential, but there had to be more than that. Tight budgeting and smart spending alone would not solve the problem—not nearly.

Initially, Kaplan was not sure what to do. He worried about the financials, of course, but the larger question was how Virginia Mason could distinguish itself in a highly competitive marketplace. It was not as though patients did not have alternatives—very good alternatives, in fact. In his thinking, Kaplan kept returning to the issue of quality. The two landmark IOM reports—*To Err Is Human* and *The Quality Chasm*—were fresh in his mind, having been released within the past year or so, and he had taken the messages of those documents seriously. Virginia Mason had a history of pursuing quality, particularly under Kaplan's predecessor, Roger C. Lindeman, MD, who had worked with Berwick and Paul Plsek on quality initiatives back in the 1990s. And Gary Kaplan had always believed Virginia Mason delivered high quality care: the finest in town. Was that still the case? How could he know for sure? He kept turning the questions over in his mind: *What would truly distinguish us in the marketplace? What would make us special? What would make us great?*

Whatever path he chose, Kaplan knew it would require a level of internal change that would surprise, and upset, many people within the organization. When the board asked him in late 2000 what they could do to help him, he suggested eliminating the long-standing Virginia Mason practice of electing department heads and the CEO. Though he himself had been elected, Kaplan knew that he would need to make tough, unpopular decisions, and he wanted department heads to have the courage to carry out those decisions without worrying about reelection. The reaction to the board's decision to eliminate elections was predictably turbulent: Some physicians threatened to start a doctors union, while others derided Kaplan for turning around and eliminating the very system that had put him in charge.

It soon became clear that Kaplan wanted to change the VMMC culture in a fundamental way. Historically at Virginia Mason—as at most major hospitals—doctors were kings of the hill. The institution and all major decisions revolved around the physicians.

"I used to pride myself in talking with candidates for jobs about this being a physician-driven place," recalls Kaplan. "A great place for doctors—physician driven, physician led." It was always, he says, about "physician, physician, physician." But now that he held the CEO position, he was adopting a different point of view. Yes, Virginia Mason needed to be a great place for doctors, but patients had to come first.

This cultural shift was not easy. As a doctor himself, Kaplan had recognized from day one that many of his fellow physicians would have difficulty adapting to the new approach. Early on, Kaplan organized a physician-only retreat where doctors did not hold back: Emotions were raw. They had always lived under a certain set of rules, and now those rules were changing. "There was a lot of mourning, in a sense, for what was past," says Kaplan. And it became clear that a new deal was needed—an explicit compact—an understanding of what the doctors could expect from Virginia Mason and what Virginia Mason could expect from the doctors. With the guidance of a skilled consultant, Jack Silversin, Kaplan and the physicians began creating a compact that Kaplan considers a foundational element of the Virginia Mason change journey. The essence of the deal for doctors was simple, as Kaplan put it: "'As a doctor I am entitled to patients because I work with a group. I'm protected from worry about business decisions because there are administrators and physicians who also have some business training, and I'm autonomous because I'm a professional.' That didn't sync up with where we needed to go. In some ways, that's what the mourning was about."

The new compact—worked out over many months—calls for the organization "to foster excellence, listen and communicate, educate, reward, and lead" while it calls for physicians to "focus on patients, collaborate on care delivery, listen and communicate, take ownership, and embrace change." With the compact, doctors went from being independent operators to being team players; from practicing the way they chose to practicing evidence-based care. Some physicians preferred the old way and left for what they considered greener pastures, though the overwhelming majority stayed.

Everyone in health care offered rhetoric around the notion that the patient was at the center of the universe, of course, but most places, Kaplan knew, mirrored Virginia Mason's physician-centric culture. As he worked with the board at putting together a strategic plan for the medical center, with the system under a microscope, it was immediately clear that "everything was designed around the doctors, the nurses, the staff."

Kaplan vowed to change that. The VMMC strategic plan, completed in the fall of 2001, was represented by a pyramid placing the patient at the top, above everything and everyone else. The language of the plan was clear: "Everything we do is ultimately to improve [the patient's] health and well-being. . . . Our vision is to be the quality leader in health care. . . . In all that we do our patients come first."

Gary Kaplan and his leadership team had established a goal. What they had not yet done was figure out how to get there. It was not as though Kaplan hadn't been trying. For years, his intellectual curiosity had propelled his engagement as a leader in several national professional associations. He knew key players in medicine throughout the country, and he had visited dozens of hospitals. As he considered what direction to take he thought, "Somebody must have this figured out." But the more he combed through the literature and his own contacts the clearer it became that no hospital had cracked the code of how to improve quality and safety significantly and at the same time control costs. It seemed incredible that with all the talent and the enormity of the brainpower in American medicine no one had yet found the solution.

In late 2000, Gary Kaplan's colleague, Mike Rona, president of VMMC, returned from a trip and excitedly told Kaplan he had met one of the country's leading quality experts during an airline flight. John Black had recently retired as a quality official at Boeing, Virginia Mason's Seattle neighbor, and he and Rona had engaged in a lengthy conversation about quality. Black had surprised Rona when he told him that the model for much of Boeing's quality improvement efforts was Toyota, an automobile manufacturer. Black said that Boeing was hardly alone—that a number of U.S. manufacturing companies had adapted the Toyota Production System (TPS) as well. Black himself had helped implement the Toyota system at Boeing, and, on numerous occasions, he had visited Japan to study the Toyota techniques. Black gave Rona a copy of his book, a slim, ninety-four-page volume titled *A World Class Production System,* which explained the Toyota approach. Rona read it and thought, "Finally, a method to match our aspiration." Rona told Kaplan he thought they should meet with Black so that Kaplan could hear from him firsthand. Kaplan read the book and found it compelling. Central to the Toyota system, Black wrote, is "the principle of stopping work immediately whenever a problem arises. Toyota production equipment stops automatically whenever abnormalities occur. Workers halt the line when defects are suspected. This prevents defects from proceeding any further into the system, and also helps identify the causes of problems by halting the line as soon as a problem is identified."

"The premise of the book is you can do twice what you're doing today with the same resources and create a higher quality, defect-free product," says Kaplan. "Anybody that tells me that—I'd at least like to hear more."

When he and Rona met Black for breakfast in March 2001, Black told them about Boeing's success with the Toyota Production System and he informed them that other companies he was familiar with—including Genie in Seattle and Wiremold in Hartford, Connecticut—had also used the system effectively.

After meeting with Black, Kaplan and Rona did some additional research and learned that the Toyota Production System was among the premier management systems in the world. Its essence was to eliminate waste—what the Japanese called *muda*—and Kaplan knew firsthand that waste in health care was at epidemic proportions (the elimination of waste in the manufacturing process—waste of time, movement, energy, money, etc.—was so central to the Toyota approach that it was also sometimes referred to as "lean" manufacturing, or, simply, lean: doing more with less). Kaplan also liked the Toyota effort to identify best practices and standardize work.

By early April, Kaplan was ready to discuss the Toyota Production System with the Virginia Mason executive leadership team, including the medical chiefs and vice presidents. Kaplan asked everyone who would be attending the gathering to read Black's book first. The meeting was held on March 26 and 27, 2001. Gary Kaplan had been CEO for just sixteen months. During that time, he had made some significant administrative moves, but he had also alienated a fair number of his colleagues who mightily resisted change. Now he had gathered the top three dozen people from the hospital to give them a primer on how the Toyota car company manufactured its vehicles. Depending on the players, this approach would be seen as audacious, visionary, or loony.

Kaplan introduced John Black, who explained how Boeing used the system to increase efficiency and quality while driving out waste and reducing costs. That Boeing, a highly respected Seattle company, had used the system certainly gave it credibility in the eyes of many at the meeting. Yet there was a certain sentiment that "we don't manufacture cars, we treat patients"—in other words, it's fine for manufacturing processes, but our work bears no resemblance whatsoever to an auto assembly line. Ironically, when Black and others first brought the Toyota system to Boeing, the airplane engineers said: "But they manufacture cars—we build jets and the two have nothing in common."

Wisely, Black had persuaded a couple of people to agree to join the meeting by telephone, including Art Byrne, the CEO of Wiremold in Hartford. By 2002, the time of the meeting, Art Byrne had had twenty years experience in working with lean, Toyota-style production, first within a General Electric lighting division, and, lately, at Wiremold, a manufacturer of wire management products for the electrical industry. Byrne recounted how, when he told associates at the company that he wanted to dismantle the Wiremold production area, they thought he was crazy. But the impact was dramatic. Wiremold came to be viewed as a particularly successful example of lean thinking. Sales, wages, and profits rose significantly. With the Toyota approach in place, the company quadrupled in size and operating income rose thirteen times, all within eight years. Eventually, Byrne sold the company, which had been valued at $30 million when he took over, for $770 million.

Via speakerphone, Byrne told the Virginia Mason gathering that he saw clear parallels between manufacturing and health care. "It's about improving all your processes to eliminate waste and make the value stream flow through your organization," he said. "Whether it's a hospital or an insurance company or a manufacturing company, every business is built on a series of different processes. Hospitals are no different."

In retrospect, Byrne sees that making progress with lean can be much harder in hospitals than other types of companies. "It's one of the most fiefdom-driven businesses I've ever come across," he says. "You've got to go through eight different fiefdoms—the blood lab, the X-ray lab, the admission people, the nursing units, the OR—and none of the fiefdoms talk to each other very well, and they don't coordinate anything very well." The problems in hospitals "aren't doctor problems, they're process problems," he says.

Also joining the meeting via speakerphone was Carolyn Corvi, vice president of Boeing, and one of the true stars of the company. Corvi was in charge of manufacturing the Boeing 737 series of jets, the company's bread and butter in the commercial aviation field, and she, like Art Byrne, possessed significant experience and credibility in the area of lean and the Toyota system. She had nearly thirty years experience at Boeing, and she told the assembled Virginia Mason team of how she had taken teams to Japan to study the TPS. Corvi had been so impressed with the system that she had gone so far as to adopt the Toyota moving assembly-line model to Boeing, a radical departure from past practices. The move was daring but proved highly successful, resulting in less waste, higher quality, increased speed, and higher profits, cutting 737 assembly time in half from twenty-two days in 1999 to eleven days in 2005.

Finally, Colin Fox from Genie Industries in Redmond, Washington, joined the discussion by speakerphone and echoed what Byrne and Corvi had said. Fox said something else that was intriguing: that the Toyota Production System allowed capable people to perform with excellence. In other words, employees need not be geniuses: Capable, dedicated people, working within the Toyota system, were capable of great work.

"The key was Carolyn and Art Byrne," Kaplan recalls. "For them to say, 'We've tried this in these two industries and it's been phenomenal.'" During the meeting, without its being forced, the message emerged: Whether it was the manufacture of airplanes, electrical molds, or small tractors, the Toyota system helped reduce waste, increase efficiency, and build in quality. Now the question hung in the air: Could it do the same in health care?

Gary Kaplan decided he and his team needed to see the Toyota Production System in action. Art Byrne generously agreed to host a large Virginia Mason contingent at Wiremold. "We spent a couple of days with them," recalls Byrne. "They were a very smart group of people. We showed them how we organize our processes, how we think about them, manage them, and what measurements we use. And we tried to relate what we were doing to health care." Byrne sought to show that although he was moving a piece of steel through a process, moving a human being through a somewhat comparable process was not really all that different; that, in fact, there were many more similarities than differences.

Kaplan was taken with it all, but perhaps what impressed him most was the enthusiasm of the employees. The Toyota system empowered each worker to become a quality overseer, and the workers derived great satisfaction from their roles. Several told Kaplan how much they enjoyed working there—though they had not at all felt that way under the old system. For Kaplan and the great majority of his team this was their first experience in a factory and it took some effort to get comfortable observing a manufacturing process. But they quickly saw past the mundane nature of manufacturing; they saw a remarkable efficiency, even an elegance to the flow of work. They saw crisp, clean steps along the way; they saw the absence of waste: waste of motion, time, and materials. And they saw the result of this process, namely, data showing the incidence of flaws at near zero. They also saw the economic results: the production of profitable products. And they saw workers engaged and energized.

Although the trip to Wiremold and a similar visit to Genie, a Seattle neighbor, were informative, Gary Kaplan was told by Corvi and Byrne that seeing the Toyota Production System at its source in Japan could provide a vision unlike any other. The folks from Boeing had found it deeply valuable, and Kaplan was convinced it was an experience that could teach and inspire his senior leadership group. As part of the exploration into the Toyota production methods, Kaplan and his team took classes in Seattle in lean thinking, the philosophical core of the system. It was arduous work—hours of reading and classroom time for his top thirty or so people in addition to their normal workload. But Kaplan could see a growing sense of enthusiasm and excitement among his team.

So he made a decision: He would take the top people at Virginia Mason Medical Center on a two-week journey to Japan to experience the Toyota system firsthand. It was, to say the least, an enormous gamble on Kaplan's part, but it was one he felt compelled to take. "We've got to go," he thought, "because unless we go, we'll never know—and we run the risk of passing up the greatest potential opportunity in the history of the organization."

"It was a gamble, but it was an *educated* gamble," says Kaplan. "We'd talked to Carolyn [Corvi] who'd led five or six teams from Boeing to Japan. We'd talked to the people at Genie, we talked to Art Byrne at Wiremold, we talked to John Black extensively. So we knew somewhat what we were going to see there."

When Kaplan disclosed his plan internally, the reaction was decidedly mixed. Some people thought it a stroke of genius, others an act of lunacy. Squarely in the later category was Fred Govier, MD, one of the most respected surgeons within Virginia Mason (who would later become chief of surgery). When the Toyota approach was first introduced, Govier and many other physicians were taken aback. Recalls Govier:

It first came out that this was the new direction of the organization, and it was all going to be about processes and standard work and people were not the same as cars but there were a tremendous amount of similarities. As a surgeon, the last thing I wanted to hear about was standard work. I was taking care of patients with complex problems and the thought we were going to learn something from an assembly line that made automobiles was just way out there for me.

The more Govier and some of his colleagues reflected on this—and quietly talked about it around the hospital—the more they came to the conclusion that this path could mean "the downfall of Virginia Mason."

Govier did not participate in the first trip to Japan and when he was asked by Kaplan to go on a subsequent Japanese mission, he was reluctant. He saw the Toyota system as "taking bright, innovative people and making them assembly-line workers." He was discouraged by spending on another group trip to Japan while a budget squeeze was preventing clinicians from buying new equipment and some doctors were leaving for better pay elsewhere. Govier heard the grumbling from colleagues: "They're going to drive this place into the ground wasting all this money sending people to Japan to learn how to build cars."

With this sort of internal reaction from influential clinical leaders, Kaplan had no intention of making his plans public, but a disaffected employee leaked it to the press, and an article appeared in the *Seattle Times* a couple of weeks before the trip:

> For the past year, Virginia Mason Medical Center has been nipping and tucking to cut costs, so employees wonder why the hospital is paying for executives to go to Japan to learn to think lean.
>
> To better implement a cost-cutting program, the medical center . . . is paying for its top 30 executives to go to Japan for a two-week training session. . . . Hospital officials didn't say how much the trip will cost.

Some employees are furious, calling the expense egregious from a company dedicated to a low operating budget. They say jobs have been cut and morale is poor because of low staffing levels.

"'Outraged' is *not* an understatement," said one employee who wished to remain anonymous. Said a former employee: ". . . this is what makes you think there's no decency left in the administration there."

As part of a four-year strategic plan, Virginia Mason has dedicated itself to "Lean Thinking," a program to help businesses cut waste and become more efficient. . . .

Groups of nine to 12 doctors and staff members attend mandatory workshops to examine everything from how long a patient waits for an appointment to the amount of paper used in offices and waiting rooms.

The article was embarrassing, of course. If the story's references to low morale and outraged employees wasn't enough, the notion that doctors were forced to sit through sessions in which the amount of paper used in waiting rooms was discussed—well, it all seemed ridiculous on its face. Who wanted to be part of such a circus? Not surprisingly, some doctors approached Kaplan and said they would prefer not to go on the trip. Some considered it a waste of time, others were embarrassed by the whole notion of it. But Kaplan told them it was important that everyone share the experience together and he reminded dissenters that the trip was all about finding better ways to care for their patients.

In 1902, a man named Sakichi Toyoda invented an automatic loom with a remarkable innovation: If any of the threads in the loom snapped, the loom would stop automatically. Broken thread, of course, would make for defective fabric and Toyoda's invention stopped the production process and allowed defects to be repaired before they were woven into the fabric. Typically, fabric was inspected after it had been woven and defects discovered only then, after much loom time, thread, and effort had gone into the process. Although this after-the-fact inspection identified some defects, it resulted in enormous waste of time, resources, and money. Toyoda's loom, however, increased production and decreased defects and was thus far more profitable to operate than other looms. As Gary Kaplan stood in the Toyoda Museum in Nagoya, Japan, watching Sakichi Toyoda's loom operate, he felt humbled. Toyoda had created this manufacturing marvel nearly a century earlier; the profits from this modest start eventually gave birth within the Toyoda Automatic Loom Works to an automobile company that would blossom into the largest in the world. More than that, though, was the notion that the philosophical basis for the loom foreshadowed the philosophical platform of the car company. In watching the loom operate, Kaplan was seeing the kind of continuous quality improvement Don Berwick had discovered from W. Edwards Deming decades earlier.

Gary Kaplan found the museum to be a tour de force. "The entire history of the Toyota Production System was right there for us to see. You could see the constant evolution in improvement. We say, 'I want it 100 percent right today!' But Toyota has been at it since 1902 and they continue to make breakthrough progress year after year. It takes time."

At Toyota's Motomachi production facility in Toyota City, Kaplan had a similar experience. From the catwalk just above the production line he watched as each vehicle approached a station, the appropriate parts would suddenly appear on the line in a fishbone: the various components—doors, engine, windshield, and so forth—met the car as it moved steadily along. Every tool necessary appeared at the point of use; everything came together as though choreographed by some manufacturing genius with artistic flair. On this very production line Toyota produced one completed, defect-free car every fifty-seven seconds!

Kaplan was struck by how immaculate the factory was—nothing even remotely like the traditional image of industrial operations. "It was like watching a symphony," Kaplan recalls. "Everything totally synchronous and you wonder what health care would be like if it actually looked like that."

Members of his team were equally impressed. Charleen Tachibana, vice president and chief nursing officer, could not believe how focused the workers were on quality. "Seeing another industry focus on quality to that extent and then seeing health care I felt shameful," she recalled. "Watching the line I could see they spent more time and energy and thought on a piece of metal than we do on our patients. I was embarrassed."

Upon returning to Seattle, some doctors bristled at the notion of standard work, feeling that it demeaned them. Standard work, they said, was a kind of robotization of medicine and thus a terrible mistake. These changes were not easy for doctors who had been trained in a culture of independence; who had been promised an implicit bargain—that if they succeeded at medical school and in their rigorous training as residents and fellows they would be given the freedom to practice as they chose; to heal the sick in the way they had been taught by outstanding practitioners. An essential part of this bargain was that the rules of the game would remain unchanged. But Gary Kaplan was blowing it up.

Some doctors feared a kind of robotization of their profession, but Kaplan had seen in Japan that, far from treating employees as robots, the Toyota Production System provided each worker with immense power. The system was based on the idea of continuous incremental improvement. Under TPS, there were no silver bullets, no huge sweeping solutions. Rather, there were dozens, and then hundreds, and then thousands, and tens of thousands of small improvements day after day after day—*continuously*—that improved quality. It was not up to management alone to foster ideas for improvement, nor was it the exclusive province of a quality department. It was the job of *every* worker; and, at Toyota, workers took this very seriously—so seriously that employees at Toyota came up with *hundreds of thousands of improvement ideas each year*—and the majority were adopted.

In Toyota City, the Virginia Mason contingent broke up into teams of five or six, each team assigned to work with a *sensei*, a Japanese advisor who had mastered TPS. Robert Mecklenburg, the Virginia Mason chief of medicine, led one of the teams along with Charleen Tachibana, the subteam leader. One evening, they were meeting with their *sensei* and explaining that they needed more space for operating rooms at Virginia Mason but could not figure out how to add them in the most efficient manner possible. Dr. Mecklenburg and his team spread a layout of a particular section of Virginia Mason on a table for the *sensei* to study. The *sensei* pointed to a waiting room and asked: "What is that?"

"A waiting room," Mecklenburg replied.

"Who waits there?" the *sensei* asked.

"Patients," Mecklenburg said.

"What are they waiting for?"

"The doctor."

There was an intensity, a seriousness to the *sensei*'s questioning. Mecklenburg was not at all sure where this was going. The *sensei* asked more questions, zeroing in on the waiting area. How long did patients wait? About forty-five minutes on average, Mecklenburg told him. How large is the area? the *sensei* asked, looking down at the floor plan.

"About 300 square feet," he was told.

"And all of the patients in the hospital wait in this room?" the *sensei* asked.

Oh, no, Mecklenburg said. This was just one of many waiting areas. There were comparable spaces throughout the medical center in one department after another. The *sensei* wanted to know how many such waiting areas there were. Mecklenburg wasn't sure, but thinking about all the departments spread across the campus, he guessed there were maybe a hundred such waiting areas.

It was as though the *sensei* had confronted an unexpected, deeply offensive cultural violation of some sort. He lowered his gaze and looked steadily at Mecklenburg.

"You have a hundred waiting areas where patients wait an average of forty-five minutes for a doctor?" He paused and let the question hang in the air, then he asked: *"Aren't you ashamed?"*

It was a kick in the stomach for Bob Mecklenburg, who had devoted his life to healing and caring for his patients. And at that moment the answer was yes, he was ashamed. The shame was in treating patients so shabbily as to make them wait; in wasting so much space throughout the medical center for waiting—an activity without any value added to patients at all. It was an activity that was wasteful in an almost pure form: It wasted space, wasted time for patients and their families, and reduced the productivity of all the patients who were missing work or school.

"In the American medical culture the doctor is the chief and people wait for the doctor and we think it's perfectly okay, but this was a real smackdown," Mecklenburg says. "Because he was right and it helped us see it in a totally new way. Because the reality is when you . . . ask the docs why is the wait so long, they will tell you, 'We're running behind because we've had a couple of emergencies today,' but the reality is that they've had a couple of emergencies every day for twenty years. Why not factor that in? Build it into the system and plan for it?"

Late at night, working with the *sensei* in a conference room at the plant, Mecklenburg and his team were going through quality improvement work, but the *sensei* was unimpressed. "You can do much better so do it again," he said. He advised them to have "big eyes, big ears, and small mouth. Sit here one hour and watch [the production system] and come back with what you see."

No employee power was greater than each worker's ability to make the decision—entirely on his own—to halt the production line. Of all he witnessed in Japan, the thing that struck Gary Kaplan more forcefully than anything else was the practice of stopping the production line to correct imperfections. This was authentic continuous quality improvement in action and the ultimate in employee empowerment.

As Mike Rona, the president of Virginia Mason, put it: "They gave all the power to the worker; this guy installs steering wheels—he's not the plant manager or engineer or regional director or president of Toyota Japan—he's the guy who installs steering wheels and he has the power to stop that line any time he identifies a defect so it does not reach the customer."

The Virginia Mason team watched as a car moving along the line arrived at the station where a worker was to install side panels. He seemed to have some difficulty, and as the clock ticked—and the car continued moving—he calmly reached over and pulled a cord. When he did so, yellow lights flashed and the line slowed until it was barely moving. It seemed only seconds later that a small team of supervisors rushed to the station to discuss the issue with the worker. As they talked, one reached out and pulled the cord again, stopping the line altogether, and red lights flashed. Within two to three minutes, the team had figured out the problem, solved it, and restarted the line. With their own eyes they had seen a potential defect eliminated before it could get to the car's owner. When a worker has comparable trouble in the medical world, Kaplan thought, usually somebody comes and chews his head off. But here, the worker is encouraged and supported. "Every worker in a factory of 1,050 workers, making 350 cars a day, every worker is empowered to stop the entire production line, rather than pass a defect down the line," marveled Kaplan. "What we saw was an unbelievable demonstration."

Gary Kaplan's reaction was almost immediate: "*We need to do this.* There's got to be an application here in health care." He vowed, upon returning to Seattle, to replicate that system; to empower all employees to take responsibility for quality.

As the team left Japan, Kaplan was exultant. The trip had revealed something new and extraordinary to his team. It had shown them a new way of doing things; a new way of creating the kind of quality care their patients deserved. When he had taken over Virginia Mason Medical Center, Kaplan had said they must change or die. If they were to change, they would have to focus on quality, but he had not been sure how to achieve it. Now he had a method.

Back in Seattle, the skeptics were ready. "You guys are nuts," one doctor said to his colleagues. "You drank the Kool-Aid." Others, appearing incredulous, asked plaintively: "What *happened* over there?" Other doctors tersely dismissed those who had been on the trip: "Why don't you go back?" they suggested. Some, upon hearing a few specifics of the Toyota system, replied: "Over my dead body."

It was not an entirely unreasonable response. These doctors had gone through enormously rigorous training over many years, and Gary Kaplan was saying that the lessons of better care were to be found on the floor of an auto assembly line. But there were also doctors who wanted to know everything about the trip; they wanted to understand this mysterious thing known as the Toyota Production System and how it might apply at Virginia Mason.

Gary Kaplan estimated that about 10 percent of the docs were in the former camp, and about 10 percent in the latter. The other 80 percent sat back and watched, saying, as Kaplan put it: "'Let's just ride this one out and see what happens.' A lot of them believed that it was just a management fad-of-the-month kind of thing." The most pointed reaction, of course, was from a wide variety of clinicians who simply did not understand how the Toyota system could have any application in a hospital. They argued that people were not cars; that every patient was different, and that to engage in some sort of assembly-line medicine was, well, ridiculous.

Mecklenburg said that was flat wrong. He told *Today's Hospitalist* magazine:

> The unique human interaction between provider and patient is not the target of any of this. Surrounding that very special and highly variable interaction are all sorts of production processes. . . . The time I spend talking with the patient and their family about diabetes is value-added. But if part of the interaction with the patient is spent looking for the records—that is a production issue. That is something that can be the subject of lean thinking.

The equation, said Mecklenburg, came down to "evaluating what's important to the patient, what adds value to patient care, what doesn't add value"—the very definition of waste—"and then eliminating the waste."

The key for Kaplan and his team was engaging the Virginia Mason community quickly in the effort to apply Toyota principles to the organization. Almost immediately upon returning to Seattle, Kaplan made two key decisions. First, he announced a no-layoff policy. No worker, he declared, would lose his or her job as a result of efficiencies achieved by the TPS. This guarantee was a crucial step aimed at calming the organization. If he was to enlist all workers in a drive to find efficiencies and eliminate waste, he wanted people to feel free to do that without fearing that their good work on waste reduction might eliminate their own jobs. Kaplan's second move was to institute a stop-the-line program like the one on the Toyota factory floor. Every hospital employee was empowered to "stop the line" if they encountered a situation in which a mistake with a patient could lead to harming that or any other patient. Every staff member became a safety inspector, charged with watching for threats to a patient's well-being and sounding a patient safety alert whenever a patient was in danger. The call would bring a response team to assess and resolve the situation promptly. After the event had passed, the team would drill down in an effort to understand fully why the threat had occurred and, in some instances, alter procedures to head off such incidents in the future.

This would not be easy to implement because it was directly contrary to the long-standing culture in medicine, not just at Virginia Mason but everywhere. Doctors are in charge. Doctors make decisions and their decisions stand unless overruled by a more senior physician. Other than that, for the most part, clinicians are there to support the doctors' decisions. Further, other patients are none of my business. When the new program was announced, many clinicians, particularly nurses, technicians, and junior physicians, expressed concern that if they raised an issue they could be ostracized or punished. It would take guts for a nurse, for example, to stand up and say she believed harm would come to a patient if the doctor did what he was planning to do. During the training process, the staff was told that a patient safety alert (PSA) could be called for many reasons: defective equipment that would harm a patient or fail to register accurate information (thus endangering the patient); medication mistakes; an inexperienced doctor (usually an intern or resident) doing a procedure incorrectly; a simple procedure that suddenly develops complicated and unanticipated challenges; and inappropriate practitioner behavior.

Two examples illustrate how the PSAs improve quality and safety and, at the same time, serve as a powerful force to alter the physician-centric culture of medicine.

In one case, a number of doctors who had referred patients for procedures were deeply concerned about the quality of outcomes. When these doctors discovered that one physician was responsible for a disproportionate number of complications, they got together and called a PSA. The chief of the specialty division responded immediately, and the doctor in question was taken off-line, that is, placed on administrative leave. This was no ordinary event. In fact, the doctor was one of the most senior at Virginia Mason. He was experienced, well-respected, and productive. The idea that a man of his background and stature could be taken off-line was stunning to the Virginia Mason community. To his credit, the doctor accepted the action without complaint. He said that if his outcomes were below those of his colleagues, he wanted to know it and try to understand why. There was a bit of mystery to this particular case: The record showed that many of this doctor's procedures went beautifully and had high-quality outcomes while others were clearly subpar.

Cathie Furman, senior vice president, was in charge of overseeing PSAs and she and a number of colleagues went to work trying to untangle the data to see whether there was any kind of clue. A statistical expert soon discovered an unmistakable pattern. Typically, this doctor would perform one procedure a day, the results of which were nearly always of high quality.

But there was a glitch. Within the department, doctors took turns being on call for emergencies and these would inevitably be the second procedure of the day. Given the complexity—and often the length of these high-risk procedures—a second one in a day was an enormous load to carry. The statistician found that in virtually every case of poor outcomes, the occurance was in the second procedure of the day. Here was a doctor performing high-quality work when refreshed and rested, but whose sub-par outcomes were all (or nearly all) the result of fatigue.

The protocol was changed so that the doctor on call would not have a regularly scheduled procedure during on-call day. Thus, when emergency cases arrived, the doctor would be fresh, well-rested, and ready to take on the job.

This particular PSA served two important goals. First, of course, it solved a serious problem and resulted in a better, safer system of conducting high-risk procedures. But there was another goal achieved as a result of this case, albeit inadvertently. This PSA reverberated throughout Virginia Mason because it was dramatically contrary to the nature of the culture. Historically at Virginia Mason, and at the great majority of hospitals throughout the country, events such as this are only whispered about. Hospitals routinely conceal mistakes even though it is clearly in the patient's best interest for mistakes to be put out in the open, examined, and learned from. Yet, every day hospitals across America work to hide mistakes. They do so to protect the reputations of doctors and nurses and pharmacists. They do so to protect their own reputations. They do so to avoid negative news coverage and potentially expensive malpractice litigation. Only in the rarest of circumstances is a senior doctor taken off-line. It was not a case where a junior person—a nurse or tech or first-year intern—had been disciplined for messing up. This had been one of the highest-profile people within the medical center and thus sent an enormously powerful signal throughout the organization that patient safety alerts are serious business; that this was not about politics or hierarchy or the old-boy network; that this was, purely and simply, about the patients; about protecting patients and doing whatever was necessary to provide the highest possible quality of care.

A second PSA involved a cancer patient scheduled for chemotherapy. For this particular chemotherapy agent, there was a specific standard of care requiring both a urine test (to make sure the urine reached a certain alkaline level) and an echocardiogram (to make sure the patient's heart was strong enough to withstand this potent form of chemotherapy). When the nurse received a written order for the treatment, she noticed that the two tests had not been completed. She assumed this was a simple oversight on the doctor's part and she called him to point it out. Surprisingly, the doctor responded sharply to her and ordered her to proceed with the chemotherapy. His attitude was conveyed strongly: *I am the doctor, you are a nurse. Do what I tell you to do.*

This type of encounter has happened countless times in medicine, and in the vast majority nurses have yielded to the greater stature of physicians. But not this nurse, not this time. She phoned the chief of cancer services and explained the situation. As much as anything, she wanted to make sure that her understanding of the standard of care in this case was correct. The chief confirmed that, in fact, she was absolutely right, and he called the chief of cancer services at the medical group where the doctor worked.

That should have been the end of it. The doctor should have been grateful that his mistake was avoided and the patient cared for in the appropriate manner. He should have thanked the nurse for making sure he did not harm a patient. Unfortunately, he took a different approach. He picked up the phone, called the nurse, and began shouting at her for what she had done. *How dare you call the chief of the department? How dare you cause me embarrassment?* The nurse did not hesitate: She called the chief of the cancer division and told him exactly what the doctor had done. The chief immediately called a PSA and the doctor in question was taken off-line. The chief made it amply clear that this sort of abusive behavior toward a colleague would not be tolerated; that the nurse had, in fact, made the correct call on the standard of care; that the nurse had protected the patient and served the patient well; that we are about the patients and not egos. To get back on-line, the doctor was required to study the standard of care more intently, sign up for an anger management class, and apologize to the nurse. When he had done these three things, he was permitted to practice again. When the matter was settled, senior hospital administrators personally visited the nurse on the hospital floor to praise her actions in front of her colleagues. Word of that spread instantly throughout the hospital.

The result of this case was that a patient had been protected and a doctor forced to learn his business more fully. But beyond that, another immensely powerful message was sent throughout the medical center—that whoever you are, if you fight for the safety and quality of patients, you will be respected, listened to, and protected. This sent a crystal clear signal throughout the hospital that management would back employees—of every rank—who did what they thought was in the best interest of a patient. And further, that there would be zero tolerance for any doctor who mistreated any other employee in any way.

Five years after the patient safety alert system was initiated, Cathie Furman, RN, MHA, senior vice president of quality and compliance at Virginia Mason, teamed up with Robert Caplan, MD, medical director of quality, to write an article in the *Joint Commission Journal on Quality and Patient Safety* (July 2007). In that time, it had become clear that the PSA system was vastly superior to the traditional approach to quality improvement. Furman and Caplan wrote:

> At VMMC, it often took weeks or months before a traditional quality incident report even received any attention. This delay made it hard to fully understand all the facts and the root causes that had led to the original problem: the trail was long since cold. Our traditional quality incident program was also characterized by a culture of secrecy that limited knowledge of the problem to those with a "need to know." This reduced creative thinking about remedies and limited the opportunity to broadly leverage safety lessons.

Furman and Caplan acknowledged that the open atmosphere fostered by the patient safety alerts could expose Virginia Mason to "legal action and negative media coverage," but, they added, "we believe it to be the right thing to do for our patients. . . . We believe that failing to report, recognize, or act on safety problems is an unacceptable breach of duty to our community." Their conclusion was that of all the Toyota inspired changes at Virginia Mason, PSA proved to be "the single most important tool to make our care safer."

When the PSA program was initiated—just two months after the team returned from Japan—there was angst that they might be overwhelmed with hundreds of insignificant complaints. But the concern that the system would be paralyzed proved unfounded. The number of PSAs in the early days was few as workers watched and waited to see what sort of reaction they received. But once it was clear that employees were actively supported for calling PSAs, the number steadily rose. In all, since the system was put in place, more than 9,000 PSAs have been called.

One of the clearest signs of the value of the TPS was its widespread acceptance throughout Virginia Mason even by physicians who had previously been among the leading skeptics. Dr. Fred Govier had certainly been in that camp, but, over time, his views evolved. Gary Kaplan asked Govier to go on a subsequent trip to Japan and, though Govier had been reluctant, Kaplan told him that in the future leaders at Virginia Mason would either work within the Toyota approach or they would move on. Kaplan told Govier that he had to decide whether the system was right for him and the best way to do that was to see it firsthand in Japan.

For several months before the trip, Govier prepared intensively with class study and extensive reading on the Toyota method. On the trip itself—when he finally made it to the floor of a Toyota factory— "it was a bit of a religious experience," he recalls. "If you walked in with no background, you'd say, 'This is neat.' But after months of preparation and knowing what to look for, you walk out of there and the more you think about it we've got systems in health care that never work and about 60 to 70 percent of stuff we do is routine stuff we do over and over and over again." He returned to Seattle and saw systems through new eyes—saw the health care system "set up to fail—it's just not well thought out."

Govier tells two stories illustrating the value of the Toyota system in health care. Some years ago, he was scheduled to operate on a patient one day when another surgeon walked into his office and breezily announced that he had already done the job. The other surgeon—Govier's partner—explained that he had been scheduled to perform the same type of operation that day, had gone in and done it, but had discovered after the fact that it was Govier's patient after all. As Govier looks back on it, what he finds remarkable is that nobody was really fazed by this. He and his associate knew a mistake had been made, but the patient got the right operation so all was well. This incident illustrates how valuable a pre-surgery time-out is. Says Govier: "I've got this patient's life in my hands the least I can do is stop and make sure I've got the right person, that I'm operating on the correct side, doing the right operation, that I have the right equipment in the room, the right personnel."

Govier vividly recalls an operation some years ago for which a very difficult situation could easily have been prevented by a pre-surgery time-out. He had a patient opened up on the operating table and was ready to install a three-piece prosthetic device in the urethra. When he called for the prosthetic device, he discovered that it was not in the OR. Worse, there wasn't one anywhere at Virginia Mason! An emergency call went out to a nearby hospital and the appropriate device was found and delivered forty-five minutes later as the patient lay on the table under anesthesia. This is precisely the sort of situation that can be easily avoided by a pre-surgical time-out, he says.

Other Toyota-inspired changes have markedly increased quality and efficiency. Smooth workflow is central to the Toyota Production System, yet a study showed that nursing workflow was anything but smooth or efficient and the result was that nurses spent far less time with patients than they wanted. Careful study revealed that geography was a major part of the problem, says Deb Heinricher, RN. "Being assigned to care for patients who are not all in one geographic area on a nursing unit [is] a major contributor to the chaos seen on many units," she says.

Using a Toyota Rapid Process Improvement Workshop, Virginia Mason nurses redesigned workflow enabling nurses to work in teams and focus on patients clustered in a defined geographic area. "The change," says Heinricher, "freed up time for nurses to more closely monitor the basics of their patients care and also afforded them the time to delve more deeply into each patient's case and thus provide higher quality care." Before the workflow redesign, nurses took 10,000 walking steps per day. After the redesign, these were reduced to 1,200. The new design allows nurses to see and hear patients more easily and quickly. It has increased patient satisfaction and helped reduce the number of patient falls as well.

At the heart of the Toyota system lies the concept of standard work. Every move along the line is standardized. When a new and better method of doing something is discovered—positioning a tool, moving an auto part—that becomes standardized. The continuous improvement within the system means that whenever a better idea is proposed it is used system wide. The overriding lesson of industrial techniques is that the greater the degree of standardization, the higher the degree of quality.

Bob Mecklenburg, the chief of medicine at Virginia Mason, worked toward the kind of standardization that would improve quality outcomes. "Evidence-based care exists for most of what we deal with in adult medicine," says Mecklenburg. That is not to say, he hastens to add, that randomized controlled trials have been conducted and revealed best practices for most maladies. That is clearly not the case. But Mecklenburg says there are other ways beyond randomized controlled trials to identify best practices. "It's all about decision rules," he says. "It's *what works.*"

Back pain, says Mecklenburg, is a good example. It used to be that when a patient at VMMC presented with back pain, he or she was given an expensive MRI. But over time, it became clear that patients with new back pain were far better off going directly into physical therapy. The treatment generally was effective and cost far less than an MRI. Mecklenburg has gone to many sources to come up with standard practices for various maladies. Randomized controlled trials indicate how to treat certain things. Specialty societies have developed standards and best practices that, in some cases, are quite useful. Personal experience provides additional standard rules. Bandolier, a Web-based service that provides analysis of treatments and leads clinicians to evidence-based guidelines, is another (essentially, Bandolier looks at medical papers and grades them based on how good the evidence base is).

The Japanese urged Kaplan and his team to think about how they made decisions, to consider carefully how systems were designed. Were decisions made with the patient uppermost in mind? *All* decisions? Were processes designed around the patient, always without exception for the benefit of the patient first? In Japan, the Toyota people talked about their focus on the customer. Their goal was to deliver a perfect, defect-free vehicle to every customer, without exception. They talked about how this would apply to health care, and one of the Toyota people said it was simple: "The patient is God."

At Virginia Mason, two examples of "the patient is God" are instructive. Virginia Mason has one of the only facilities in the Seattle area designed for the care of geriatric patients. A physician in the unit one day realized that hospital employees were working while sick with colds and flu. This had been happening for years, of course—well-intentioned doctors, nurses, and technicians who, even though they were ill, wanted to make it into work and get their job done. Previously, however, no one had ever thought much about the very real danger this posed to patients, particularly weakened elderly patients.

The Toyota system had taught the Virginia Mason team to use the Rapid Process Improvement Workshop (RPIW) tool. This technique brought a team together for from three to five days to solve specific problems. In this case, the problem was employees coming to work with the flu, often not exhibiting symptoms. A quick bit of research revealed that only about 36 percent of health care workers nation-wide get flu immunizations. At Virginia Mason, it was higher—about 50 percent. Nonetheless, about half the Virginia Mason staff could potentially distribute germs that could be dangerous, and in some extreme cases deadly, to certain patients.

The solution was arrived at very quickly: All workers in the medical center, without exception, would be required to get a flu shot. Most people reacted sheepishly, wondering why it hadn't been done years earlier. But because the health care culture is what it is—where the focus has often not been on patients first—there were objections. The Washington State Nurses Association filed a grievance concerning the fact that mandatory immunization was subject to collective bargaining. The idea that a nurses' association would place convenience or preference ahead of the health of patients spoke volumes about the health care culture.

But Gary Kaplan and the other leaders on his team had no intention of backing down. They were convinced of the wisdom of the new policy. It was a perfect example of doing what was in the best interest of the patient. After legal wrangling, the order stood: Every employee and contractor working within the hospital—anyone who might have contact, however incidental, with a patient—was required to get a flu shot or wear a mask during flu season. The message from Kaplan and the rest of the hospital leadership to anyone who balked was simple: *This is not about you. This is not about the doctors and nurses; it is about our patients and doing everything we can to keep our patients healthy and safe.* We can talk all we want about putting the patient at the top of our strategic plan, at the peak of the pyramid, Kaplan argued, but unless we act on that at crucial moments it is just talk, and meaningless talk at that.

One winter, the immunization rate was 50 percent. The next it was 96 percent, and 98 percent the year after. A few nurses unable to have the immunization (usually because of side effects or previous allergic reaction) were permitted to wear masks during flu season. A handful of others refused to get immunized or wear a mask and they were fired.

Another specific case of putting the patient first involved the treatment of ambulatory cancer patients. With the TPS training, a group involved in rehabbing the cancer center conducted some statistical work. They plotted the path taken by patients who came in for their chemotherapy or radiation treatments. Many of these men and women were among the sickest ambulatory patients cared for at Virginia Mason, yet the TPS-inspired study found that their trip to the hospital on treatment days was anything but comfortable or easy. The study found that many patients, upon arrival at the hospital, were forced to walk long distances from one building to another, and often to a third to get blood tests, see their oncologist, and then receive their treatment. Against the backdrop of the Toyota Production System, it was obvious to the Virginia Mason team that such logistics fell far short of putting the patient first.

The oncology group set about designing a new outpatient cancer center. In the new space, patients would sign in and undergo blood work a few feet from the reception area. They would then walk a short distance to their doctor's appointment. Rather than hiking halfway across the hospital campus to obtain their drugs, a satellite pharmacy was built in the cancer center, steps from where patients received treatment. Working with architects, the oncology team had created a beautifully warm and inviting space that was configured to reduce the strain of patients' hospital visits.

The final touch involved a brief collision between the old culture (docs on top) and the new (patients on top). The design of the new facility called for spacious rooms on the perimeter, each with a large window and plenty of light. Those spaces were the most desirable in the new area, and the question was what would they be used for. Would they be physicians' offices, as surely they would have been at any other time in the institution's history? Or would they be given over to patients?

If the patient always comes first, there could be no other answer. The outer spaces were designed as treatment rooms, and they were equipped with comfortable lounge chairs, reading material, flat-screen television sets, and other such amenities—all to make the patient feel as comfortable as possible during treatment. There was room for friends or family members. The staff had thought of everything.

And the doctors' offices? They were built in the middle of the floor, all small, windowless offices. With the new design, all the services patients needed were within steps of each other, including the lab, pharmacy, social work, the doctors and nurses, and the oncology infusion center. Before the new center was constructed, average lead time for patients from arrival at the hospital until the start of treatment was four hours. Since then, it has been reduced to ninety minutes. Under the old system, patients walked a distance of 748 feet. Now, it's 181 feet.

And as Denise Dubuque, the administrative director of the Cancer Institute, put it: "When a patient isn't feeling well, even walking 10 steps is a lot. This new space is designed so that all of the services come to the patient, not the other way around. It's putting the patient first."

Two years into the application of TPS at Virginia Mason, tragedy struck. Mary McClinton, a sixty-nine-year-old patient, was undergoing an invasive radiology procedure on the brain and was supposed to be injected with a contrast dye. But instead, she was injected with a toxic skin-cleansing solution. Nineteen days later, on November 23, 2004, she died.

Virginia Mason made no effort to hide the mistake or to conceal anything about the case. The day Mrs. McClinton died, the hospital made an announcement explaining that she had died as a result of a preventable error. The hospital took full responsibility. A memo from two senior physicians to the Virginia Mason staff explained what had happened. "The solution used to clean skin before and after procedures was recently changed from a brown iodine-based solution to a colorless antiseptic," the doctors wrote. The memo said that the colorless antiseptic looks "exactly the same" as the dye. "At some time during the procedure, the clear antiseptic solution was placed in an unlabeled cup identical to that used to hold the marker dye . . . that is injected into blood vessels to make them visible on X-rays." The patient suffered "kidney failure, a sudden drop in blood pressure and a stroke."

Virginia Mason announced the patient's death, disclosed that it was due to preventable error, and apologized publicly. Robert Caplan told the *Seattle Times:* "We just can't say how appalled we are at ourselves and the suffering of this patient and her family and friends. We're trying in every way we can to convey our apologies to this patient for this preventable medical error. In many ways, this open and honest communication is our way of trying to honor her." The hospital changed the way the antiseptic was applied—via a swab on a stick—to insure that it would never again be injected into a patient.

The ultimate question, of course, is whether all the work and effort to institute the Toyota Production System has been worth it. Is Virginia

Mason Medical Center a better place for it? Does it deliver safer, higher-quality care now than before? Gary Kaplan says it is an ongoing journey; that the path to full transformation is a series of countless incremental improvements. Have there been enough of those incremental improvements to make a real difference?

A number of measures and indicators are instructive. In 2004, 2005, and 2006, VMMC received a Distinguished Hospital Award for Clinical Excellence from HealthGrades, a company that measures quality. No other hospital in Washington could match this distinction. In 2005, Virginia Mason ranked first in Washington in The Leapfrog Group's quality and safety survey. Virginia Mason was the leader in implementing recommended safety practices in nearly every category measured by Leapfrog. In 2006, Virginia Mason again led the region in implementing Leapfrog's safety standards and was one of only fifty-nine hospitals in the United States to be named on the Leapfrog Group's Top Hospitals 2006 list.

At Virginia Mason Medical Center they are not ashamed. They have learned countless lessons in their journey thus far. One is that the Toyota Production System fits very nicely into health care. Gary Kaplan will be the first to say they have a long way to go. But they are on their way to a level of transformational change that is rare anywhere in the world today. And although there are constant problems and challenges, Kaplan and his team never, ever, forget the central truth of their mission: The patient is God.

8

Josie King

———∞∞———

*"They say anger can do one of two things to you. It can
cause you to rot away or it can propel you forward."*

Life was very good for Sorrel and Tony King and their four young
children. They were living in a beautiful home in suburban Baltimore, Sorrel had set aside her clothing design business to care for
the children, and Tony was enjoying success in financial services.
But everything changed on the night of January 30, 2001, when Sorrel heard her youngest, seventeen-month-old Josie, screaming up-
stairs. Sorrel raced up and found that Josie had managed to turn on
the hot water and climbed into a scalding bath. The Kings lived a
short ambulance ride from Johns Hopkins Hospital, and Josie was
admitted that night to the Hopkins pediatric intensive care unit, a
sixteen-bed facility for seriously ill and injured children. Josie had
suffered second-degree burns over 60 percent of her body—parts of

her feet, legs, chest, back, arms, and face. While Sorrel and Tony were terrified—none of the kids had ever been seriously sick or injured—they were comforted by Hopkins. Josie's pain was soothed with morphine and several skin grafts restored the most badly burned areas. As frightening as the accident had been, the prognosis promised a full recovery.

Sorrel remained at Josie's bedside night and day, spending hours staring into her eyes, profoundly grateful that something worse had not occurred. She was comforted by the very presence of her child and by an overriding confidence in the institution of Johns Hopkins Hospital. She had been told, and fully believed, that it was the finest hospital in the country, and perhaps the world; that it attracted the very best and brightest doctors and nurses anywhere. Sorrel developed a sense of awe, a kind of reverence for the medical staff. It seemed to her that every encounter with them elicited either compassion or brilliance, or both.

Every day, Sorrel saw the grave conditions faced by other children in the PICU (pediatric intensive care unit). Some of these children would not be going home any time soon. Some would not live through the week. Sorrel was humbled and deeply thankful that Josie's prognosis was so positive. After a couple of weeks her biggest concern was that Josie would grow up with scars on her feet. The idea that something bad would happen to her daughter at the hands of the Johns Hopkins professionals "never, ever, ever crossed our minds." As Josie healed during the first couple of weeks, Sorrel and Tony talked about how they wanted to get involved in helping Hopkins, perhaps by donating and raising money. They were determined to help make a difference.

After two weeks, Josie had improved significantly—enough so she would no longer need the intense attention provided in the PICU—and the doctors transferred her to an intermediate care floor for a few days before her release. Sorrel had come to know the doctors and nurses in the PICU quite well, and she would miss them. The idea that Josie would be cared for by a new team (with some crossover) concerned her a little. As they rode the elevator down to the intermediate care floor, Sorrel asked the nurse, "Are you sure we're going to be okay down here?" And the nurse replied: "Sorrel, no one has ever come back up—you'll be fine."

In the new unit, Josie continued doing well, although she developed an upset stomach and threw up a couple of times. The nurses wanted her to avoid fluids, so she was allowed only ice chips until her stomach settled.

The next day, Sorrel noticed that Josie seemed very thirsty. When someone went by with a drink she would reach or call out for it. On the intermediate care floor Josie no longer needed a central line in her chest, so that night, Sorrel was able to give Josie a real bath. As she did so, she noticed Josie sucking furiously on the washcloth. Josie was also lethargic and limp, to the point where Sorrel had to hold her up in the bath. After the bath, Sorrel laid her down in bed and was struck by how listless she appeared. "Can we call a doctor?" Sorrel asked the nurse. The nurse replied that Josie looked tired but was fine.

But she did not seem fine to Sorrel. Josie's eyes didn't look right— they were rolling back in her head in a way Sorrel had never seen before. "Something's not right," Sorrel said. "Can someone else look at her or can a nurse look at her?" Another nurse then examined Josie and found her vital signs normal. Sorrel was unsure what to do. Her instincts told her that something was wrong, but she also recognized that she was in the best possible hospital. These were gifted people who knew what they were doing. Sorrel had developed wonderful relationships with a number of doctors and nurses and she did not want to bother them unnecessarily or come across as a high maintenance mother. "I thought if they liked me they would take better care of Josie."

Sorrel was exhausted and the nurses urged her to go home for a while and get some rest. Since Tony was leaving for the West Coast the next morning, Sorrel decided she would go home to see him briefly and get some sleep. Sorrel called the hospital twice during the night; both times she was reassured that Josie was fine. But when she walked into Josie's room at 5:30 the next morning, Sorrel screamed, ran into the hall and shouted for help. *"Please come!"* she called out. *"Please come!"*

Sorrel could see that Josie had deteriorated during the night. She was not moving and her eyes had a sunken look. Doctors and nurses responded promptly. Josie had been on methadone as a way of easing her off the powerful painkillers that had gotten her through the worst of the burn pain. Now doctors theorized that her lethargy was caused by oversedation with methadone. Doctors administered a drug to reverse the effects of the methadone, and in just twenty minutes Josie had improved. Sorrel asked whether Josie could have some fluid, and she was given twenty ounces of juice. Sorrel asked the doctor whether Josie's regular dose of methadone for the day could be skipped, and he agreed. When the episode had subsided and the medical team began to drift away, Sorrel grew more worried. "Please don't go far away," she asked the doctors. "Mom," one of them said to her, "we've got other patients to see." Sorrel understood that, of course, but she was frightened and she wanted them nearby in case anything else happened to Josie. But as the morning wore on, Josie seemed better as she watched cartoons on television.

Early that afternoon, a nurse entered the room with a syringe to administer methadone. Sorrel intercepted her. "I talked to the doctor and he agreed to cancel the methadone," Sorrel said. The nurse replied that the orders had been changed.

"What do I do?" Sorrel later recalled. "I have a decision to make. Do I grab the methadone and run into the hall and scream for help? Or do I say, 'I'm in the best hospital in the world . . . '"

"She gave her the methadone," Sorrel recalls, and as she did so, Sorrel was massaging Josie's feet with the help of another nurse. Then the nurse helping Sorrel said, "Oh, a little crocodile tear." Sorell recalls: "And I look and think, *God, that's so weird—Josie had never once cried during her stay in the hospital after all she had been through and now this one single tear—one tear.* And then I looked again and her eyes were rolled way back in her head and she was totally out and I'm screaming for help and the nurse is pushing buttons and all these doctors and nurses came running in and there were metal trays and tables and chairs and carts and people ripping open things. And I remember the PICU doctor, Amal, coming in and looking up at some monitor and saying, 'What the hell happened here?'"

Josie had gone into cardiac arrest. She was rushed through the hallway and back up to the PICU while Sorrel was guided to a private room in the company of a chaplain.

Soon, shaking with fear, she was led from the room and guided to a back stairway and up to the PICU. Josie was hooked up to various machines as doctors and nurses surrounded her bed, all standing quite still. Sorrel said to them, "Everything's going to be fine, I don't care what it costs, it doesn't matter what it takes—fly in whatever surgeon we need for a transplant or whatever it takes. You did this to her—you guys are the best. *You* need to fix her so let's get to work right now."

And someone said: "We need to pray." And then Sorrel realized they were all filing silently past her, leaving her, leaving Josie.

Desperately frightened, Sorrel thought: *God ain't gonna fix this so please get back in here and please help.*

The next morning the neurologist told Sorrel and Tony that Josie was brain-dead. Her organs were shutting down and she was dying; it was just a matter of time.

Sorrel asked whether a miracle was possible.

Sorrel sat holding Josie's hand through much of the night thinking *please squeeze my hand, please flutter your eyelids, please move.*

The next day, her siblings—ages six, five and three—were brought in to say goodbye. Sorrel and Tony took turns holding her and, at 6:11 P.M. on February 22, 2001, Josie died.

They left the hospital insisting on an autopsy—and, says Sorrel, "our lives were ruined."

Initially, the Hopkins team said they weren't certain of the cause of death. They talked about the possibility of sepsis, but the real cause of Josie's death was that no one at Hopkins had listened to Sorrel. No one had listened to the one person in the world who knew the child better than anyone else. No one had taken Sorrel's concerns seriously enough to conduct a complete and thorough examination of her child. It would later be discovered that signs of trouble were everywhere: a dramatic loss of weight, severe diarrhea, declining blood pressure.

Traditionally, hospitals often instinctively conceal the truth. When terrible things happen, lawyers step in and take control and when that happens sometimes the truth is a casualty. In cases such as this one, the hospital typically goes into a lawyer-controlled bunker while the aggrieved family sues. The hospital ends up either settling or going to trial. During the proceedings, the family and the doctors typically encounter one another only in court or with attorneys present.

This story is different.

A week or so after Josie died, George J. Dover, MD, chief of the children's center at Hopkins, arrived at the home of Sorrel and Tony King, accompanied not by a lawyer but by Josie's pediatrician. Dr. Dover had phoned the pediatrician and asked to accompany her to the King's house for a conversation. On a raw, rainy February night, Dover arrived and began by apologizing to Sorrel and Tony. He told them that what had happened to Josie should not have happened.

He said he was very, very sorry. And he assured them that he had a team investigating it and that they would get to the bottom of it and figure out exactly what went wrong. "Don't tell me what went wrong because I know," Sorrel said. "She died because she was thirsty and no one listened to me and you guys gave her the methadone." Sorrel and Tony were civil with Dover, but no more. Their grief was as profound as their anger was justified. George Dover's hospital had killed their little girl.

That night, Dover said that he was setting aside every Friday afternoon at one o'clock for a phone conversation to update Sorrel and Tony on what the investigative team had learned that week. Sorrel would field those calls, which took place every week for more than a year.

"Most of those early conversations were pretty much like 'You better figure it out,'" Sorrel recalls. "I cried on the phone, used four-letter words on the phone. The tone was always angry and sad. I wasn't like totally insane crazy, but it was probably really hard on George to have to talk to me every Friday at one o'clock."

Sorrel had loved Hopkins and the people who worked there. The idea that they could make any sort of mistake seemed impossible to her. They were the best and brightest—how could they make a mistake that would cost a child her life? How was it that no one had connected the dots between the intensity of her thirst, weight loss, diarrhea, and lethargy? Sorrel was shattered. In the weeks and months after Josie's death, she would find herself sitting alone in Josie's room staring into space. Some days she was so angry she wanted to see Hopkins hurt the way Josie had been hurt. She wanted Hopkins punished, she wanted the institution to suffer. She considered going to a newspaper or filing a malpractice suit. Tony King would later tell the *Baltimore Sun:* "She was so angry that she just wanted to do whatever she could to bring down Hopkins."

During this time, Hopkins offered a financial settlement. The entire money issue troubled Sorrel. At the urging of her father and her father-in-law, an attorney, she and Tony had retained counsel and their lawyer urged them to accept the offer. Settlement papers were drawn up, but Sorrel wasn't signing. During one of their Friday phone calls, she told Dover: "We don't want the money. If you think giving us the money lets you off the hook . . . "

"The only thing more disgusting than them offering to pay money would be for us to take the money," she said later.

But their lawyer called one day and told Sorrel that if they did not take the money the only one who would benefit would be some insurance company. The lawyer urged Sorrel and Tony to take the settlement and do something positive with it. The simple logic of this argument was persuasive, Sorrel and Tony came around, and the settlement was formalized in August, 2001. In a surprising twist, the Kings felt that they should do something with Hopkins. Perhaps because she felt so deeply connected to the doctors and nurses who had initially cared for Josie (and, Sorrel, in a way) she couldn't let go. She remembered seeing children in the PICU suffering from cancer, and after talking it over with Tony, they decided they would start a foundation for kids with cancer—focused on patients at Hopkins.

Sorrel is not shy, nor does she stand on ceremony. As she and Tony were contemplating the foundation, Sorrel picked up the phone one day on impulse and called the lawyer at Johns Hopkins, Rick Kidwell. Kidwell put her on hold almost immediately, phoned Sorrel's lawyer, and secured permission to talk with her. When he came back on the phone, he apologized to Sorrel for what had happened. Sorrel told him that she and Tony were trying to figure out what to do with the money and she felt she needed to check on one thing.

"Rick, this medical error thing," she said, "what happened with Josie was just a total fluke, a strike of lightning, right? It was a one in a million, a crazy, crazy thing, right?" He replied, "Sorrel, no it was not. It happens everywhere. I see it every day." He referenced the IOM estimate of 98,000 preventable deaths per year in American hospitals. *It was not a fluke? Happens all the time? To 98,000 people a year?* Sorrel King was about as shocked as she had ever been in her life.

Sorrel plunged into researching the subject of medical errors, and it became quickly apparent to her that Rick Kidwell was absolutely right. In the course of her work, Sorrel met Peter Pronovost, MD, a patient safety expert at Hopkins. Sorrel and Pronovost bonded quickly when Sorrel discovered that his father had been the victim of medical mistakes for years when he was misdiagnosed, failed to receive the right treatment, and died.

Sorrel's discussions with Pronovost were enlightening. She was getting a tutorial from a true expert on the nature of error in medicine. During their work together, Pronovost asked Sorrel whether she would speak to a group at Hopkins, and Sorrel agreed. It was the first time she spoke publicly about what had happened to Josie and, appropriately, it was during Hopkins grand rounds in front of a standing-room-only crowd. She had told George Dover in advance that she intended to speak out in the future: "If you guys think I'm going to keep my mouth shut, you [have] got another thing coming. I want everyone at this hospital to know what happened," she told him.

She was terrified when she stood before the crowd—she had never done anything like this before—but her combined sadness and anger helped her focus and convey the raw truth of what had happened.

"I told Josie's story," she said. There was a nice simplicity to that: *Josie's story;* not Sorrel and Tony's story or Hopkins's story, or any doctor or nurse's story. Part of Sorrel wanted to get up there and "just scream at them" but, of course, that would have accomplished nothing. And she wanted very badly to accomplish something. She wanted to get their attention because she thought that if she could get through to them it might help change things; it might help prevent something terrible from happening to someone else's child. She asked for their help in solving the "epidemic" of hospital errors. She vowed not to rest "until we make something good come out of [Josie's] senseless death." The core of her message was as simple and compelling as it would always be: She urged them to learn to communicate better, to "listen to the mother, listen to the patient, listen to each other."

A couple of weeks later, Pronovost told Sorrel that he would be attending an IHI meeting in Boston, and he invited her to come with him. He thought she would be an ideal speaker at the event. At the conference, Pronovost introduced her to Don Berwick and Maureen Bisognano, and Sorrel spoke to the group just as she had at Hopkins grand rounds.

Sorrel moved gingerly into the limelight. It was not her first choice, not something she would ever have sought, but she realized that she was in a position to draw attention to errors in health care as few others could. She told the story of what had happened with Josie, and the emotional struggle she and Tony had faced:

> On top of our overwhelming sorrow and intense grief we were consumed by anger. They say anger can do one of two things to you. It can cause you to rot away or it can propel you forward. There were days when all I wanted was to destroy the hospital and then put an end to my own pain. My three remaining children were my only reason for getting out of bed and functioning. One day I will tell them how they saved my life. My husband Tony and I decided that we had to let the anger move us forward. We would do something good that would help prevent this from ever happening to a child again.

A doctor in the audience taped Sorrel's appearance, and it has since been viewed thousands of times. Many clinicians have contacted Sorrel to thank her for giving them a new perspective on their profession and to tell her that the video has changed the way they listen to patients. When Sorrel speaks at conferences, people reach out to her, hug her, hold her hand, pull her aside, and whisper to her their own stories about medical errors in their families.

Peter Pronovost told her the story of a nurse at Hopkins who was caring for a child when the mother asked to see her daughter's medical record. The nurse reacted with instinctive suspicion: *I'm the nurse, why does she want to see the record?* But the nurse recalled Sorrel's remarks at grand rounds. She looked the mother in the eye and told her she could absolutely look at the record, and after she had done so, she should feel free to ask any questions she might have. She told the mother that they were a partnership—nurse and mother—caring for the child together.

Along the way, Sorrel has come to realize how unusual the reaction of Hopkins was to the mistakes they made; how rare it was for someone in George Dover's position to come to the house and say essentially that we made a mistake, we're sorry, and let's work together and we'll fix it. "Most families aren't told the truth," says Sorrel, "and that's heartbreaking on top of all the other anguish they're going through."

There are times when she feels the safety movement is advancing rapidly; but sometimes she is jarred by what appears a lack of progress. Back in 2005, she spoke to a group of Johns Hopkins first- and fourth-year medical students and asked how many had heard of the IOM report *To Err Is Human.* To her horror, not one student raised a hand—not one—although she thinks things have changed since then.

Sorrel and Tony set up a Web site (www.josieking.org) with the mission "to prevent others from dying or being harmed by medical errors. By uniting healthcare providers and consumers, and funding innovative safety programs, we hope to create a culture of patient safety, together."

In 2005, Don Berwick invited Sorrel to the IHI Forum in Orlando and asked her to join him—along with the heads of several hospitals—on the stage when he announced the launch of the IHI

100,000 Lives campaign. One aspect of the campaign was to save lives through the use of rapid response teams (or "Condition H" for "help") in hospitals. When Berwick had finished describing the campaign, he asked whether Sorrel would like to say something.

"When I first heard of rapid response teams I was sitting on the stage with Don Berwick. My mind was going through these flashbacks to when Josie was in the hospital and I thought, *'Oh, my God, that would have saved Josie.'*"

She took the microphone and spoke of how the idea appealed to her, asking whether rapid response calls were limited to clinicians. Could a family call such a team? Would a patient be able to do so? She said she had no doubt in her mind that if such teams had existed five years earlier that Josie's life would have been saved. She said she would have called the team that night when she was frightened because Josie's eyes were rolling back in her head and she was not herself. She would have called when Josie was sucking so desperately on the washcloth. And she would have called that morning at 5:30 when she found Josie so listless. The team was there to do what the doctors and nurses had not done: to listen to her. If there had been a rapid response team at Hopkins, she said, "I wouldn't be here today and my daughter would be six years old."

Just a week after Sorrel spoke at IHI, she received a call from a nurse at the University of Pittsburgh Medical Center (UPMC) who had heard Sorrel speak at the IHI Forum. The nurse, Tami Merryman, was involved in quality and safety at UPMC and she said she had been so moved by what Sorrel had said that UPMC had decided to go ahead and create a rapid response team. "If people are able to call 911 from their home, why is this control taken away from them when hospitalized?" Scores of hospitals throughout the country have since set up such teams. At UPMC in one year they found that 69 percent of Condition H calls "would have led to potentially harmful patient situations if Condition H had not been called."

At the IHI Forum in 2007, Sorrel was asked whether she ever wonders why every hospital doesn't have rapid response teams. "I think about it every single darn day," she replied. She noted that statistics show that nearly two-thirds of the most serious medical errors are the result of communications errors. "They don't listen."

Sorrel writes infrequently on her foundation Web site blog, but when she does so it is on an issue with great meaning for her. In June of 2007, she wrote:

The thing that really continues to amaze me is the communication issue. Josie died because people didn't listen. They didn't listen to me, and they didn't listen to each other. I can't tell you how many stories I have on my computer from families who have been affected by medical errors, and there always seems to be a common thread, "They didn't listen." Correct me if I'm wrong. Doesn't the Joint Commission report that over 60 percent of all sentinel events are due to a breakdown in communication? I am not a doctor or a nurse. I am not at the bedside, and I am not an expert in the field of patient safety; however it seems to me that if people communicated better we'd all be safer. I believe in high-tech solutions. It is where we are heading, but wouldn't we get more bang for our buck if we communicated better?

Every year, hundreds of thousands of Americans lose family members to medical errors. Most suffer in silence, finding their own private ways to deal with their grief, but an increasing number are actively engaging in the new quality movement with the hope of effecting change. Sorrel is one particularly compelling example, but there are many others—including Armando and Victoria Nahum. Within a one-year period, three members of the Nahum family were afflicted with hospital-acquired infections: Armando's father, wife, and son. His seventy-five-year-old father suffered a mild heart attack in Rochester, New York, and acquired an infection in the form of bacterial pneumonia. Fortunately, he recovered in a matter of weeks.

Victoria Nahum suffered terribly for several years until it was discovered that she had been infected with bacteria during breast augmentation surgery six years earlier. Bacteria had evidently been living within Victoria's chest wall for years, and the apparent and likely cause was a medical error when the implants were inserted. Victoria went through a hellish period, but she survived.

In September 2006, Armando and Victoria received the terrible news that their twenty-seven-year-old son, Josh, who was living in Loveland, Colorado, and working as a sky-diving instructor, had been injured in a parachuting accident. He had broken his femur and fractured his skull. The femur was quickly repaired by insertion of a titanium rod, but his skull was a far more serious issue. A neurosurgeon drilled a hole in Josh's skull to drain fluid built up around his brain, and within a couple of weeks he was slowly improving. During this time, he was struck with a staph infection that was caught quickly and treated successfully with antibiotics. After a few weeks, Josh was transferred to a nearby rehabilitation facility and seemed on the road to recovery. But less than a week later he grew nauseated and his fever reached 103 degrees. Josh had developed another, more serious bacterial infection in the fluid around his brain. No sooner had this been diagnosed than Josh fell into a coma and stopped breathing.

He was placed on a ventilator and another hole (the fourth) was drilled in his skull to relieve pressure. But the surgeon made an alarming discovery: Somehow the pressure of the bacteria had pushed part of Josh's brain into his spinal column, permanently damaging his spinal cord. The doctors told Armando and Victoria that Josh now faced a life as a quadriplegic permanently attached to a ventilator. Two weeks later, however, at age twenty-seven, Josh died.

Armando was disconsolate, but Victoria had to act. She found it incredible that three members of the same family had contracted hospital-acquired infections in such a short period, and she set about doing some research. She found that such infections were as common as they were preventable. She discovered that every year an estimated 1.7 million Americans were victims of health care acquired infections—4,600 *per day!* The more she learned, the more profound was her sense of shock that this was allowed to happen throughout the medical world.

Eventually, a time was arranged for Armando and Victoria to meet with officials at the hospital where Josh had been treated. They flew to Colorado, and when they arrived at the hospital (they prefer not to disclose the name), they were greeted by the CEO. He told them that his hospital's infection rate stood right at the national average. Armando and Victoria were taken aback by this. Was he saying this proudly? Was he thinking this would somehow help them heal?

The CEO ushered them into a conference room and introduced them to a group of doctors, nurses, and other health care professionals. But there was one person, a woman, seated next to the CEO whom he did not introduce. Armando at once thought this peculiar, but somehow in the pit of his stomach he knew who she was. He went over and introduced himself. She told him her name. And what do you do, he asked? She said she was the hospital's attorney.

Any hope of an honest conversation, any anticipation that the truth would be discussed in an honest way, evaporated for Armando and Victoria. Armando pointed out that he and Victoria had come alone—that they felt no need for legal representation. This wasn't a legal mission, after all. It was about the death of their son; about understanding and honesty and truth.

It's not uncommon for hospitals to pay careful attention to legal exposure. Many hospital administrators and physicians live in fear of malpractice suits. And a vocal minority has insisted that the new quality movement will not succeed until there is comprehensive reform of the nation's malpractice statutes. It is true that mistakes can and do result in lawsuits, but refusing to be transparent in anticipation of change in American laws is akin to waiting for Godot. Courageous hospital leaders are taking a stand and committing to transparency in the belief that it is their obligation to disclose errors, apologize to those harmed, and make sure that the same mistake never harms another patient.

Sister Mary Jean Ryan, CEO of the Baldrige award-winning SSM health care system, pointedly addressed the liability issue at the launch of the IHI *100,000 Lives* campaign. Her advice to hospitals fearing malpractice suits: "Suck it up." In other words, transparency is the right thing ethically. It is the most powerful driver of quality improvement, and *not* to be transparent out of fear of a lawsuit is self-defeating. And there is no evidence that hospitals and systems that have adopted a transparent approach have experienced a boom in malpractice suits.

"The liability system scares people and is expensive," says Berwick. "But it's not going to change in the short run and we have to simply have the courage to say, 'I'm not going to let a badly de-signed tort system keep me from protecting my patients and the only way I can protect my patients is transparency.'"

Lucian Leape argues that when mistakes are made they must be disclosed and the institution and or individual must apologize to the patient or patient's family. "The ethical duty to heal is linked to trans-parency," observes Leape. Leape has invested significant time study-ing the reactions of clinicians and families in the wake of an error, and he believes that from the clinical standpoint there is a powerful need for "honesty, openness, and apology." When an error harms a pa-tient there are two victims, he argues: The patient and the caregiver. Patients are not only harmed physically but emotionally; they also suffer a loss of the enormous trust placed in the clinician. And the clinician, says Leape, often suffers profound "shame, guilt, and fear."

From his work, Leape believes patients desire three things in the wake of an error: To know the truth about what happened, to receive an apology, and to be assured that steps are being taken to prevent similar mistakes in the future. This last point is particularly important, says Leape, because "knowing that changes were made so that others will not suffer gives a positive meaning to the patient experience—their suffering was not in vain." Caregivers, he believes, want patients to know that the harm was unintended and that the caregiver "was trying hard to do the right thing." They also want the patient to know they feel ashamed and have a deep desire for forgiveness. Leape refers to what he calls the "malpractice myth"— that honesty with a patient about a mistake increases the chances of being sued. Leape says that evidence shows the opposite is true.

Courageous leaders throughout the country are willing to publish their data for the sake of openness and improvement, even though many fear it could be used against them in litigation. The Wisconsin Collaborative for Healthcare Quality includes twenty hospitals and twenty-one physician groups (many of them competitors) who publish comparative data based on a common set of measures they collectively developed out of a conviction that such an approach is in the best interests of their patients. The Harvard hospitals in Greater Boston have adopted an explicit policy; it states that when an error occurs clinicians must "tell the patient and family what happened; take responsibility; apologize; explain what will be done to prevent future events." (Unsurprisingly, given the Harvard language, Leape was an influential member of the committee that formed the policy.)

Like Sorrel—like all families victimized by a medical error—the Nahums faced a choice: They could stew in their anger or they could try to move forward constructively. They chose the latter course, and have since established the Safe Care Campaign—Stopping Hospital Acquired Infections. It has gained widespread attention for the issue of hospital-acquired infections. Victoria has been interviewed by a variety of television and print reporters, and she has spoken at a number of medical meetings. Their Web site (safecarecampaign.org) provides consumers with important information about how to reduce the likelihood of infection during hospitalization or outpatient care.

Berwick admires the Kings and Nahums for becoming grassroots quality activists, and he recognizes that they pay a steep price for their involvement in the movement. "They get exhausted by repeating and repeating their stories," he says. "These are people who also need to heal—we shouldn't have to rely on them so much. We don't rely on the victims of plane crashes to testify about the need for safe planes."

Sorrel sees activism among an increasing number of patients and families harmed by errors as a powerful addition to the movement. Although hospital administrators and senior clinicians are certainly capable of ignoring the quality movement when it speaks about transformational change or about applying industrial quality techniques in hospitals, how does one ignore Sorrel King? There are countless stories of devastating harm to patients throughout the country—a parent hurt, a child killed. To hospital leaders and doctors and nurses there is nothing theoretical or policy-based here. This is reality, and for these clinicians who care so deeply, it is the ultimate nightmare. And these instances of harm are getting the attention of health care stakeholders everywhere.

"I think things are changing," Sorrel says. "I really do." She says she sees signs in many places that there is much more awareness that clinicians must communicate more effectively, listen more closely, and work together in partnership not only with one another but with patients and family members as well.

Sorrel hates being away from her children, but she accepts as many speaking requests as she is able. "When I stand in front of an audience and come home and look at my computer and talk with these people, I think Josie's story is changing the health care industry person by person. I think it's changing things for the better. I absolutely believe that."

9

The Learning Journey of Jönköping County, Sweden

———— ⌘ ————

*"We find ideas we like and we immediately
go back to Sweden and do them."*

There are no nonstop flights out of Boston's Logan Airport to Stockholm, which forces Don Berwick to pick his travel poison in the form of a connection through Newark, JFK, or even O'Hare. With waiting and connection time, it takes him a good nine hours to get to Stockholm from his IHI office in Cambridge, and then an additional three-plus hours by train to reach the southern Swedish city of Jönköping. The lengthy journey notwithstanding, Berwick loves coming here because he sees this as a place doing potentially breakthrough quality improvement work—among the finest anywhere.

What is so great about it? Berwick says it starts with a passionate leadership troika and its insatiable appetite for new improvement ideas. "There's nothing they won't try to do if they think it will improve care," he says. It is "the largest scale systemic endeavor focused on all systems improvement" that he knows of.

Sweden as a whole scores impressively on international health comparisons and is ahead of the United States, for example, in key measures such as life expectancy and infant mortality, where it ranks at the top in the world (with Japan and Iceland)—less than half the rate found in the United States. Cancer deaths per thousands are lower in Sweden than in the United States (155 per hundred thousand vs. 175 per hundred thousand). A Commonwealth Fund survey found that among nineteen countries where deaths "could have been prevented by access to timely and effective health care" the United States ranked last and Sweden tied for fourth. Although 90 percent of doctors in Sweden rely on technology—generally Electronic Medical Records—to help in their practice, in the United States only about one quarter use such technology.

And, for all the quality they produce, Berwick loves how they control costs. The idea that a free-spending socialist state is tossing money indiscriminately at health care is not even close to the reality here. In fact, even as Sweden's outcomes are generally better than those in the United States, care in Sweden costs less than half the price of care in the United States ($2,825 per capita versus $6,100). The U.S. devotes 16 percent of gross domestic product (GDP) to health care; Sweden devotes 11 percent.

Berwick likes the Swedish system generally, but he has a particular fondness for Jönköping because in a nation delivering quality care Jönköping is the star. When Sweden's twenty counties (each of which manages the county health system) are compared on a variety of eleven quality measures, Jönköping consistently ranks at the top. Jönköping is the best of a very good system and, most impressively, it is steadily getting better. Berwick knows how difficult it is to effect change in health care, and he credits the Jönköping leadership with real courage for the transformational work they are doing. And, Berwick being Berwick, he praises their courage specifically, not generally, noting their courage to aim so high, to take on a learning journey and find solutions throughout the world, to compare results, and to make changes when discovering that something does not work.

Jönköping County lies about equidistant from Stockholm to the north and Copenhagen to the south. The county sits at the southern tip of Lake Vättern, the second largest lake in the country, marked by a landscape lush with spruce, pine, and small farms. So pristine is the lake that it serves as the drinking water supply for many towns along its coast.

In Sweden, health care is funded out of county tax revenues and every citizen is completely covered from birth to death. Care is administered by each of the twenty counties, and Jönköping, with three hospitals, thirty-four health centers, and forty-seven dental clinics, provides care for 330,000 residents in thirteen communities.

On the surface, the pace of life, particularly the pace of work, is quite different in Sweden compared to that in the United States. Work in Sweden is done calmly, without the frantic nature that sometimes characterizes work in the United States. And yet the apparent serenity—a defining cultural characteristic—is somewhat misleading in health care, at least in Jönköping County. For although the county's official aspiration—to provide its citizens "a good life in an attractive county"—has an appealing modesty to it, beneath that surface lies a fiercely competitive desire to be nothing less than the finest health care delivery system in Sweden and beyond. The CEO of the Jönköping County Council (the county's governing board), Sven Olof Karlsson, puts it this way: "If you are a leader you must think as a sportsman—you must love to win, you must hate to lose. We want to be the best."

The leadership threesome Berwick alluded to is comprised of Karlsson; Göran Henriks, chief of learning and innovation; and Mats Bojestig, MD, chief medical officer. The three men, separately and together, have been on a learning journey for two decades. Sven Olof Karlsson has served as CEO of the county for twenty-five years, and his evolution from a single-minded focus on controlling finances to advancing the quality cause has enabled the Jönköping effort. (A former Swedish paratrooper, Karlsson was once dropped into the northern wilderness and forced to survive on his own—which, someone joked, may be ideal preparation for running a modern health care system.) Karlsson has worked with Göran Henriks for two decades, and Henriks has served as the day-to-day leader of the learning journey. Dr. Bojestig brings a clinical perspective without which none of the improvements would be possible. Of the three, Karlsson is a sort of father figure to Henriks and Bojestig. He is affable and he chooses his words carefully. Bojestig, a youthful man with a sunny personality, has the mind of a scientist. When the Jönköping team engages with others in the world of quality, Henriks is clearly their point man.

As Berwick observed, this troika will quite readily try anything, and they have experimented with just about *everything*. Many hospitals or health systems focus on a particular approach—the Toyota Production System or the Baldrige process, for example—but in Jönköping not only have they tried many improvement techniques but they have made productive use of each one.

The quality improvement techniques, programs, and ideas they have tried include the Balanced Scorecard; the IHI Breakthrough Series; IHI's Pursuing Perfection; the Baldrige process; W. Edwards Deming's system thinking; and both IHI *100,000 Lives* and *5 Million Lives* campaigns (during which they did all six improvements in the first campaign, all twelve in the second, and then added urinary tract infections and falls on their own). They have adapted industrial quality techniques from the Swedish truck manufacturer Scania and worked in partnership with Paul Batalden and his Dartmouth team on microsystem improvement. They have sent a large team to every IHI Annual Forum since 1996 and have traveled to learn from Brent James in Salt Lake City, Uma Kotagal and her team in Cincinnati, the folks at Kaiser Permanente in California, and many, many more. And a good number of the leading quality improvement hospitals in the United States have sent delegations to Jönköping to see their work firsthand.

The soul of the Jönköping improvement effort lies within a learning center called Qulturum that may be unique in the world of health care. Qulturum is set in a beautifully refurbished, modest-sized building on the leafy campus of the Ryhov Hospital in Jönköping. (The building formally served as a staff kitchen and dining area for the county psychiatric hospital.)

In his often understated fashion, Göran Henriks describes Qulturum as "a place where people can just meet and reflect." It is, of course, much more than that. Like Henriks himself, it is a combination of characteristics: retreat, think tank, training center, classroom. Under Henriks's leadership, Qulturum's mission is to provide education, training, and a place to discuss and debate ideas, all toward improving the quality of care. Hundreds of the county's frontline caregivers, as well as administrators and clinicians, have been trained there in quality improvement.

At Qulturum, the learning focus is on a series of broad topics— "learning and innovation, access, prevention and self-care, cooperation and flow, clinical improvement, patient safety, medication, and good finances." The Qulturum belief is that these are the keys to the best possible quality. Qulturum has no administrative or line responsibility within the Jönköping system (it is funded with 0.003 percent of the county health care budget—about $2 million last year). Thus,

Henriks is free to find and develop good ideas and spread them throughout the system.

Through his work at Qulturum, Göran Henriks has become one of the world's best-known thinkers in the new quality movement. He has studied psychology, worked as a child psychologist, and earned an MBA, but he is really an intellectual amalgam—teacher, student, philosopher, motivator, innovator, visionary, and leader who brings to health care a philosophical sense that seasons his teachings. He is also a reflective man with a philosophical bent. Sustainable change in health care, he says, is to some extent rooted in human emotion. People do not change because they are ordered or coerced—"People change because of love for something—a deep emotional involvement."

Although financial incentives are very much in vogue in American health care, there are very few in Jönköping. "We don't believe in financial incentives on a personal level," says Henriks, revealing a cultural difference between Sweden and the United States. "We have very motivated employees. You put fifteen years of your time learning something, you can't stand to see poor performance. The best incentive for our employees is being the best."

When he is asked whether a burning platform within an organization is needed to trigger transformational change, he ponders the question briefly and then quietly replies in a tone that conveys a sense of assurance: "The burning platform is always *inside* people."

About the pace of change: "We think we should move as fast as possible and as slow as possible."

On motivation: "Motivation to improve comes from knowledge and inspiration, not orders."

He quotes Gandhi, defining leadership as "a group of people going in the same direction by the will and the conviction of their own."

On change: "There are two ways to make change. One way is to threaten people and the other is by giving them space and allowing them to see the possibilities—to see if their eyes open for change."

Underneath his sometimes Zen-like exterior, though, Henriks is a relentlessly energetic searcher of ideas to improve care in Jönköping County. "If any system shows better results then we go and try to copy that system," he says. "We test any good idea."

Their determination to learn can sometimes lead to bold moves. When the IHI/Robert Wood Johnson Pursuing Perfection program was announced and hundreds of hospitals and systems were competing for inclusion, the folks from Jönköping went to IHI and worked a deal that allowed them to pay a fee and be included in the project. Henriks, Bojestig, and Karlsson recognized Pursuing Perfection as a unique opportunity to learn not only from IHI but also from the other participants in the program whom the Swedes knew would be on the cutting edge of improvement efforts in the United States. They wanted to figure out how to create a measurement for how their system was doing—a metric that would allow them to measure the overall quality of care. Working with the IHI team, Henriks, Bojestig, and Karlsson identified ten indicators that define system quality; for example, mortality, cost per capita, patient satisfaction, quality of life. This measurement was rudimentary when they started, but they had at least taken a stab at it—few other systems had even attempted it—and they would work to refine it over time.

Karlsson, Henriks, and Bojestig exhibit confidence, but no arrogance. Quite the opposite. The learning journey reveals much about the character of the Jönköping quality improvement effort because it is based on an implicit declaration: *We do not have the answers. We are not the best. We are not as good as we want to be. We need to improve and we need help doing so.* This embodies the unpretentious nature of the Jönköping approach to quality improvement. Perhaps it derives from the calm, self-effacing nature of the Swedish culture. In contrast to major academic medical centers in the United States, the absence of arrogance is striking. In the United States, there are hospitals, board members, clinicians, and administrators who challenge the notion that they should make an effort to learn about quality. The very suggestion offends them; affronts their unshakable sense of grandness about themselves and their institutions. This hardened crust of hubris is to be found nowhere in Jönköping County.

In 1995, at a small quality conference in Stockholm, Henriks and Bojestig met a member of the IHI board, the former Birthday Club member Vinod Sahney. The two Swedes eagerly listened as Sahney talked about a new improvement method outlined in a recent book by Robert S. Kaplan (of the Harvard Business School) and David P. Norton. Their "Balanced Scorecard" approach took a broad view of managing an organization toward quality and suggested that "financial measures tell the story of past events." These were inadequate for "guiding and evaluating the journey that information-age companies must make to create future value through investment in customers, suppliers, employees, processes, technology, and innovation." What most attracted Henriks and Bojestig was the balanced scorecard's approach calling for collecting data and measuring an organization's progress from four distinct perspectives: learning and growth, business process, customer, and financial. On the first page of their book, Kaplan and Norton cleverly make the case for their approach:

> Imagine entering the cockpit of a modern jet airplane and seeing only a single instrument there. How would you feel about boarding the plane after the following conversation with the pilot?
>
> Q: I'm surprised to see you operating the plane with only a single instrument. What does it measure?
> A: Airspeed. I'm really working on airspeed this flight.
> Q: That's good. Airspeed certainly seems important. But what about altitude. Wouldn't an altimeter be helpful?

A: I worked on altitude for the last few flights and I've gotten pretty good on it. Now I have to concentrate on proper airspeed.

Q: But I notice you don't even have a fuel gauge. Wouldn't that be useful?

A: You're right; fuel is significant, but I can't concentrate on doing too many things well at the same time. So on this flight I'm focusing on airspeed. Once I get to be excellent at airspeed, as well as altitude, I intend to concentrate on fuel consumption on the next set of flights.

The authors note that skilled pilots are able to "process information from a large number of indicators to navigate their aircraft. Yet navigating today's organizations through complex competitive environments is at least as complicated as flying a jet. Why should we believe that executives need anything less than a full battery of instrumentation for guiding their companies?" The balanced scorecard is about performance measures that guide management, just as an instrument panel guides a pilot. The scorecard measures financial performance, of course, but it is much broader than that; it also measures business functions related to customers, internal processes, as well as learning and growth.

Henriks, Bojestig, and Karlsson thought the scorecard approach was a particularly apt fit in Sweden in the way it looked beyond finances to other factors, and they began to lay the groundwork for putting it in place.

Indicative of their appetite for various quality improvement approaches, at the same time they were initiating the Balanced Scorecard, the team was working with the Baldrige structure. The Malcolm Baldrige Award, named for a former secretary of commerce of the United States, is given to companies and organizations considered outstanding in various areas from leadership to strategic planning, from customer and market focus to measurement and analysis. Henriks and his colleagues applied for the Swedish Baldrige as early as 1992 (and then again in 1998, finally winning it in 2002).

"It was a very important experience because we then understood that the concept of processes was something we didn't have within our system," says Henriks. "When we started to work with this in '92/'93, we started to understand that the clinical result depended on how we worked in the patient process and not in the employees process."

Early on, it became clear that there were serious quality problems within the Jönköping system. One of the three county hospitals had a colon cancer surgical performance level well below the others, for example. When shown these results, surgeons were taken aback. They had always believed they were performing at an advanced level clinically, but they had never before been measured. Faced with measurable results for the first time ever, they were thrown into an uncomfortable, unfamiliar, moment of confusion and self-examination.

"They saw the differences between the hospitals—they got very afraid," recalls Henriks. "They had to have meetings during half the year to find a method to really support each other to change the work patterns so they could get the higher level every time in all three hospitals. It took three months before they were there to talk with each other about this problem."

Later in the 1990s, physicians discovered they could reuse expensive cardiac pacemakers (battery-operated devices that help the heart maintain a regular rhythm). But the second time around, the devices needed expensive retrofitting and maintenance. As part of his quality push, Henriks studied this practice and discovered that the expense of repairing used pacemakers exceeded the price of a new one, but many within the system were so convinced of the wisdom of pacemaker re-use that it took Henriks two years to convince them—with hard data—that they were wrong. These sorts of incidents frustrated

Henriks. He felt as though he was working on quality in a scattershot fashion rather than systematically, and he realized he did not know *how* to work on it in a systematic fashion. And that realization prompted them to mount their global learning journey. In December 1996, Henriks and Bojestig flew to New Orleans for the Eighth Annual IHI National Forum on Quality Improvement in Health Care. There they found a community of people who shared their mission and vision. They took in dozens of seminars, discussions, and speeches during three days of the conference. The teachers and speakers included Berwick and Batalden, Blan Godfrey and Lucian Leape, Maureen Bisognano, Brent James, Jack Wennberg and Gene Nelson from Dartmouth, Diane Miller from Virginia Mason, Dave Gustafson, Vin Sahney, Jim Roberts, and Allyson Ross Davies from the Birthday Club.

More than a decade later, Henriks vividly recalls the conference. "I remember *everything*—Dr. [Larry V.] Staker from Intermountain talked about work with diabetes, Brent James talked about clinical improvement work—both coming back to need for good statistical process. It was the first time I had a deeper understanding of statistical method."

He and Bojestig heard the keynote address in which Don Berwick talked about how new ideas are adopted in various settings and why it often takes so long to adopt even the best remedies. (Berwick noted, for example, that from the time citrus was found to be a remedy for scurvy to the time it was adopted as the preventive policy in Britain's Royal Navy was 264 years!) Berwick read E. M. Rogers's book *Diffusion of Innovations* and talked about Rogers's definition of the "characteristics of the people who adopt innovation." Berwick explained that

> the fastest adopting group . . . is called *Innovators*. They are distinguished from the rest of the population by their venturesomeness,

tolerance of risk, fascination with novelty, and willingness to "leave the village" to learn, as it were. Rogers calls them *cosmopolite*. They belong to cliques that transcend geographical boundaries, and they invest energy in those remote connections. Innovators who were studied in traditional Colombian villages left on trips to cities about 30 times a year, while the average resident left 0.3 times a year.

Berwick was describing Henriks and Bojestig! They were, indeed, cosmopolites: citizens of the world, comfortable and adaptable anywhere. They were constantly "leaving the village" to go out and find new ideas for quality improvement. Henriks and Bojestig found it a feast for the mind—one session after another with thoughtful analysis and ideas that might well be applicable in Jönköping. Henriks's affable, outgoing personality enabled him to connect with many people at the forum, including Paul Batalden, whom the Swedes met for the first time and who would be an advisor for many years to come. "We were so enthusiastic," recalls Bojestig. "It was a real rush."

It was one thing to have Henriks and Bojestig enthusiastic about change, but nothing would be accomplished in the system without enthusiasm from county CEO Sven Olof Karlsson. Although Henriks and Karlsson had a close and trusting relationship, it was one thing for Henriks to tell Karlsson about what he had seen and learned and quite another for Karlsson himself to experience it. The following year, Karlsson joined Henriks and Bojestig at the IHI forum and pronounced it "fantastic." Quality, he could see, was a direct result of standard work derived from evidence-based care.

It's most important if you want to change health care [says Karlsson]. For me—it's like you met God or something. I became convinced that this must be the way we should change our health care system. We were at a small seminar, and people who talked to us at the seminar—they have done the work. They didn't talk about what we should do—which we often are doing in Sweden. They had *done* it. And they had the results. It was so concrete.

I became so convinced. When you have been at the cinema, and you want to go home and tell your wife what you have seen, it's not so easy. You can be very excited—you have seen a very fine movie—but you can't explain it because the person who you're explaining it to doesn't have the same frame as you have.

Karlsson declared that the following year they would travel to IHI with their full leadership group of a dozen or so people. They would split up and cover different classes and, at day's end, they would convene and each person would then recount to the group what he or she had learned (and that is in fact what they have done every year since).

Not all health care leaders are like Uma Kotagal—burning with desire for quality improvement at age twenty-seven, and burning even more at fifty-seven. Many have come up through a traditional system where the leader's main responsibility was to watch the money—and health care has always been a business where watching the money was something akin to solving a Rubik's cube while simultaneously playing a chess match.

Karlsson came from this traditional mold; indeed, Henriks jokingly referred to his friend and boss as Mr. Budget. Before becoming CEO, Karlsson had been chief financial officer of the county and thus had long viewed the world through a financial lens. That continued when he became CEO—not at all atypical of CEOs of major medical centers throughout the world. "For years I never was satisfied," Karlsson says. "I was always negative. I told them they must do more, work harder." But the learning journey changed Sven Olof Karlsson.

"I asked myself, 'What have you told them today? You have told them that they must work much harder with their finances—their budgets. You must work much harder with access.' It was always a bad message and I asked myself, 'Who wants to work in a system where the leader is never satisfied?'"

A shift to focusing on quality by no means meant that Karlsson gave up his ingrained sense of fiscal discipline. In fact, he made sure that underlying the improvement effort is an unbreakable law: Improvement work in Jönköping County must never create additional costs. "You must *always* have control over finances," he says. "If you do not have control over finances you cannot work on quality improvement." Financial stress and chaos drain energy and creativity from an organization, he says, and only with strong finances can the attention and energy of an organization focus on quality work. Over time, the Jönköping leadership defined their improvement strategy as "based on three principles: Learning is key to improvement; improvement needs to be broad and deep; and improvement must be both bottom-up and top-down."

The learning aspect is the soul of the Jönköping journey and it involves lessons large and small, philosophical and technical. It involves tracking data to measure quality continuously. The idea of broad and deep improvement is a rejection of the idea of projects or pilot programs which, Henriks and his colleagues believe are too limited. In Jönköping, they define broad as improvement that reaches across the system, covering all patients, while "deep signifies that as many people as possible, at every level of the system, are engaged in the improvement, increasing the likelihood that the improvement will become permanent."

The top-down idea is part of the learning process. In practice, Henriks, Bojestig, and Karlsson comb the world for ideas they think might work in Jönköping. They bring those ideas back and put them to the test. Then comes a key learning component: The front-line clinicians whose job it is to implement the changes determine whether the new technique works and how it might have to be tailored to greater effectiveness. Although the team is keen to bring back basketloads of ideas, they are respectful of the views of front-line workers. Ideas are never forced down through the ranks, never pushed upon the front lines.

The three principles—learning, broad/deep, and top-down/bottom-up—have informed their work going forward. An important result has been a leveling of the hierarchy: a cultural shift that embraces the value of all contributors no matter what their position. This was revealed particularly vividly when a team from Kaiser Permanente visited Jönköping to study their work. John August, the executive director of the Coalition of Kaiser Permanente Unions, is one of the senior people within the labor union representing workers at Kaiser and is therefore acutely sensitive to issues of hierarchy in the workplace. He says he and his Kaiser colleagues were struck by the significant cultural changes achieved in Jönköping in terms of equality among team members. "We walked into a meeting in Jönköping and we could not tell who was the doctor and who was the nurse, who was the tech, who was the medical assistant," recalls August. And in the world of health care, that is rare, indeed.

The guidelines also led Henriks and colleagues to focus intensely on clinicians on the front lines of care, and this led them to develop a strong working relationship with Paul Batalden, Gene Nelson, and their colleagues at Dartmouth. Batalden and his team had developed a new approach to working on the front lines of medicine, which they characterized as microsystems. Batalden had been studying improvement in health care for many decades and the Dartmouth team had come up with an approach that cut through all the layers of bureaucracy directly to the point at which clinicians cared for patients. This was the microsystem. As the Dartmouth project defines it: "Microsystems are the building blocks that form hospitals.

The quality of hospital care can be no better than the quality produced by the small systems that come together to provide care." A microsystem is "the place where care is made; quality, safety, reliability, efficiency and innovation are made; staff morale and patient satisfaction are made."

If they learned and improved both top-down and bottom-up—and if they were truly successful in spreading innovation throughout the microsystems—then they would have a chance to achieve their mission, which Karlsson defines in simple, aspirational terms: "We have to do the right thing every time every day for every patient."

The learning, broad/deep, top/bottom—all of what they have gotten from IHI and others—all comes together around a patient called Esther. So much of what they have learned has been applied to caring for Esther—to improving the processes of care that enhances her quality of life.

Who is Esther? On the surface Esther is a fictional patient, the name for a project to remake patient-centered care. More deeply however, in Jönköping County Esther is, metaphorically, everyone—she is all patients, and Henriks, Bojestig, and Karlsson are ever mindful of her, as are all the other caregivers in the county. Esther has become their passion, their obsession. Although Esther is not a real patient—she is a composite created by Bojestig and others—they very much think of her as real because, in fact, there are thousands of Esthers for whom they provide care every day.

Esther is a woman living alone, and she has not been well lately. She is getting along in years and in recent days, her breathing has grown labored and the edema in her legs is severe enough to prevent her from lying down at night. She does not want to burden anyone, but she knows she needs help and she calls a home nurse who has visited before. The nurse is very caring. She takes an oral history, examines Esther, and tells her that she needs to see her general practitioner. Because the stairs are too difficult for Esther to negotiate, the nurse calls an ambulance and Esther is transported to the doctor. She is examined and there is more oral history—the same questions she has already answered from the nurse and a few from the ambulance attendant. The doctor tells her she needs to get to the emergency room. He summons an ambulance, and Esther is delivered promptly to the ER where an assistant nurse examines her and asks her a series of questions (the same questions asked earlier). After a wait of about three hours or so, a physician comes in and examines Esther and asks her a series of questions (the same as before). He orders X-rays and admits Esther to the hospital. It is now six-plus hours since Esther phoned the home-care nurse. Esther is brought up to the ward where she is greeted by another nurse who takes her to her room and asks her more questions (the same as before).

That Esther is anything but a living, breathing person is hard to discern when speaking with Bojestig. He talks about her quite carefully, as though she is a beloved patient he centers his practice around. It is as though Bojestig, Henriks, and Karlsson have brought back their many lessons to Jönköping, distilled them, reshaped them, and funneled them through the system directly to Esther.

The idea to create Esther came out of the learning journey—a conference Bojestig and Henriks attended in Stockholm where they heard IBM consultant Inger Sandnes discuss business process reengineering. After her presentation, Bojestig and Henriks spoke with her at some length and it became clear to them that they could use a similar approach to attempt process reengineering in health care. They returned to Jönköping with a new idea—they would put their system under a microscope, study each step in the process of a patient's journey through the system, find the duplication and waste, and learn what worked and what did not work—*from the patient's point of view.*

Henriks and Bojestig thought it important to name the project for a patient who could be easily imagined and every clinician in the health service at any level could easily imagine Esther—they had seen patients like her countless times. Most important, Esther helped everyone in Jönköping remain patient-focused, which was what the project was all about.

Mats Bojestig said that when they followed Esther's care, on the first day they discovered that she had encountered thirty-five health care providers in the county in a significant duplication of services. This fragmented approach made no sense, and Bojestig saw it immediately. "Esther needs it to all fit together," says Bojestig, and he and many clinical colleagues went about redesigning the system of care.

An essential part of the Esther project was to break down silos and other barriers that separated various caregivers. Under a microscope, Bojestig and his colleagues could see the extraordinary redundancies in Esther's care; and they could also see the gaps. They observed a distinct lack of flow, a kind of stop-and-start and stop-and-wait approach that served no one. The team working on the Esther project interviewed scores of nurses, doctors, home care attendants, therapists, pharmacists, and ambulance personnel, and in the process they discovered a disturbing inconsistency in communication and coordination of care. Bojestig said that many redundant procedures slowed down her care significantly. Each person she dealt with seemed confined to an individual silo—competent in his or her own area but seemingly too little connected to the step in the process that preceded or succeeded them. Bojestig discovered that this seemed true of the home-care worker, ambulance crew, physician, emergency department, and so on. Rather than a series of individual siloed stops, Esther needed a seamlessly connected process without waste or redundancy and with an ongoing understanding of and focus on her particular needs.

Over several years, Bojestig asked the same question at each critical juncture: "What's best for Esther?" In time—just as had happened at Virginia Mason—when clinicians thought of Esther they first thought about what was in her best interest, and they came to conclusions different from those they might have reached in the past.

As part of the process, they studied flow through the emergency department and surgical units, and they discovered many instances of unnecessary delay and waste—no one silver bullet, but rather many small items that, when altered, made a significant impact. For example, they learned that everyone—save the most dire emergency cases—was treated essentially equally in the emergency department. But that didn't make any sense for a woman in her eighties suffering from a variety of issues. Thus, they created an emergency room fast track for Esther that got her into treatment much sooner. This was part of creating a work process that seamlessly moved Esther along, thus insuring her security while smoothing transitions and getting the right information to the right place at the right time. The Esther process was akin to taking apart an overly complex piece of machinery, finding the waste and redundancy and then reassembling it as a sleeker and much more responsive model.

This was business reengineering—a Deming approach—but it was also making process and management and flow decisions with a patient-centered mindset. In Japan, the *sensei* had told Gary Kaplan and his team that the patient was God. In Sweden, the patient was Esther. The project sought to integrate care across the system so that it would work seamlessly for Esther from ambulance service to primary care; from occupational therapists to social workers; from community clinics to nursing homes—across the spectrum of care.

Over several years of working on the Esther Project, important results emerged. Waiting times were reduced for referral appointments to both neurologists (from eighty-five days in 2000 to fourteen days in 2003) and gastroenterologists (from forty-eight days in 2000 to fourteen days in 2003). These were meaningful achievements as well as symbolically significant. One of the major complaints about the Swedish system concerned lengthy waiting times to see specialists and to reduce the wait so dramatically was a breakthrough achievement. Esther helped keep many patients healthy enough at home as outpatients so that they avoided hospital stays. Heart failure patients improved so much that their hospital stays declined by nearly a third (3,500 to 2,500).

But the biggest breakthrough was that the project had improved the process so significantly that it resulted in a 20 percent reduction in hospital admissions between 1998 and 2003 (9,300 admissions to 7,300). This sort of reduction in hospital admissions was all but unheard of anywhere in the world. Part of the success was due to improved management of the population's health—of all those Esthers out there. But part of it was due to the reengineering microscope, which had revealed that doctors and patients had found clever ways around the previously interminable waits for specialists. Let's say Esther needed to see a neurologist. As an outpatient it might, under the old system, have taken her up to three months to get an appointment. But if her primary care doctor admitted her to the hospital—using some bureaucratic excuse—she would see a neurologist the next day. Thus, patients were being admitted as a way to see a specialist more quickly. By revising the scheduling process—forcing out all the waste they could find and restructuring office visits to specialists so that nurses could play a larger role and take some of the volume from the doctor—they were able to cut wait times dramatically.

When Berwick learned of these results he was exultant. Focus on the patient led to more efficient and safer medication protocols as well as crisper communication between links in the chain (an essential element to improvement because numerous studies had shown that poor communication was a leading cause of errors). There were other improvements, of course, including stronger IT support all along the chain of care, for example. But it was clear that Bojestig, Karlsson, and Henriks had achieved an *integrated* system of care for Esther.

In the process, the county has achieved a dramatic reduction in falls by elderly inpatients. Research found that nearly one third of county residents sixty-five and older experience a fall at home, and 10 percent of those result in serious injury. A combination of Qulturum training for clinical teams, safer flooring, and better lighting reduced falls at one nursing care location from as many as twenty in some months to fewer than five.

Asthma had been an increasingly serious pediatric problem in Sweden for a couple of decades. Although just 2 percent of children suffered from asthma in 1980, by 2000 that had quadrupled to 8 percent. Again, waiting times were a very real problem; sometimes the wait for an asthma specialist was as much as six months! But a close examination of the work flow revealed that much of the clinical work involved with asthma management could easily be done by nurses, and only a minority of cases required the advanced skill of a specialist. A combination of nursing care and nurse-instructed home care by parents and kids reduced asthma hospitalizations by nearly two-thirds from 1995 to 2003. And acute hospital visits for children with asthma have now been reduced nearly to zero.

The surgery department at Varnamo Hospital, one of the three Jönköping hospitals, was experiencing serious waiting times—in some cases patients waited for months for endoscopy and diagnostic imaging. A careful Esther-like review of the detailed process revealed that as many as one in five procedures were not clinically necessary. Under the microscope, it also emerged that physician production was surprisingly low. A combination of increased doctor productivity and the elimination of unnecessary procedures brought the wait times down to just fourteen days.

As part of the Esther Project, clinicians sought to do everything possible to keep elderly people from getting sick in the first place, and they were able to increase the percentage of elderly residents getting flu shots from 39 to 70 in a matter of just a few years. Indeed, Jönköping has achieved significant improvement through the use of evidence-based guidelines. A variety of infections have been reduced and orthopedic care, as well as many other types of care, has been improved.

It is worth noting, in particular, progress on access. General lack of access to care, and lengthy waits for appointments, has plagued Sweden and other state-run systems for years. In Sweden, the government has pushed hard for improvement and as of 2004, 255 Jönköping teams at Qulturum had undergone study and training concerning access. The Swedish government wanted patients to be able to get a primary care appointment within seven days and, by late 2004, nearly 90 percent of Jönköping patients could do so. The system had long been plagued with lengthy telephone waits. Only 34 percent of patients in Jönköping had their calls answered within three minutes. After the Qulturum learning and training sessions, 88 percent of callers got through within three minutes. There was no magic involved in the improvement process at Qulturum; rather, a systematic, microscopic examination of the problem broke down each aspect in a search for wasted time, motion, or both. Qulturum was a place where people came to talk and reflect—a place where they were not hurried or rushed. The comfortable atmosphere lent itself to workers feeling free to discuss every aspect of a problem—slowly, carefully, completely. This approach of taking apart the broken watch and spreading out the parts on the floor enabled improvement teams to see how things really worked—and then to strive for a more efficient, streamlined way to operate. Qulturum was Zen and the art of motorcycle maintenance—broadly philosophical and microcosmically practical. The approach did not always work, of course, but in many instances it did—and with impressive results. At Jönköping's Varnamo Hospital, for example, patients waited months for ambulatory surgery, diagnostic imaging, and endoscopy. After the Qulturum learning and training, the waiting time was reduced to just fourteen days.

Don Berwick has traveled the world for thirty-plus years working on quality improvement, and he says there is no better example of progress than Jönköping. He draws an analogy between Jönköping County and health care and Toyota and automobile manufacturing. Berwick, Tom Nolan, and their IHI colleague Andrea Kabcenell wrote that at some point in the future

> maybe the shock will be just as it was in the automobile industry; an attractive product developed outside the U.S. . . . Jönköping County which has proven overall to be the highest performing of all Pursuing Perfection sites, both financially and clinically. . . . [It] has perfected its chronic disease management to achieve some of the lowest population-based hospitalization rates for asthma that IHI has ever seen.

In ObGyn, the department head says that through sustained effort most of the critical work has been standardized. "We say this is the way we're going to do it and then everybody does it," says Dr. Raymond Lenrick.

In the January-March 2007 issue of *Quality Management in Health Care,* Berwick observed that Jönköping had achieved an overall approach to quality "perhaps unparalleled internationally." He urged others to study the Jönköping approach as a model that other health care systems might emulate. Says Bojestig: "We are ready for standardization."

Excitement for continuous improvement is palpable throughout the organization. Karlsson says that one of the most heartening developments has been employees who come before gatherings of colleagues to report quality advances large and small. "They always start their presentation saying, 'I thought it was impossible, but . . . '" he says.

Perhaps most important, the culture has changed. Jönköping is now a place not only of continuous learning but of continuous improvement. It starts at the top, of course, with the teachings of Henriks and Bojestig. And Karlsson, who used to spend all his time on finances, now spends 40 percent of his day on finances and 60 percent on quality improvement. "We find ideas we like," says Henriks, "and we immediately go home and do them."

10

Kaiser Permanente and the
Future of Health Care

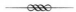

"The single most important thing that can be done to improve the quality, safety, and efficiency of health care today is to widely implement Electronic Health Records."

From an early age, George Halvorson loved to write. In high school, he edited the school paper, wrote poetry and stories, and contributed to his weekly hometown newspaper in Menahga, Minnesota. At Concordia College in Moorhead, Minnesota, he continued writing poetry, short stories, and plays. His work in the college literary magazine caught the eye of an editor at the *Fargo Forum* in North Dakota, and Halvorson was hired to work part-time for the paper which, in turn, led to a *Wall Street Journal* internship in 1968.

After college, Halvorson was working toward an MBA at the University of Minnesota, when he responded to an ad placed by Blue Cross of

Minnesota for an underwriter. Unfamiliar with the insurance industry at the time, Halvorson thought the term *underwriter* meant *assistant writer*. When he showed up at Blue Cross for his appointment, the interviewer could not help but howl at Halvorson's misunderstanding; but when the laughter had died down, it just so happened that the company had an opening for a writer in the communications department.

Thus did George Halvorson begin a career in health care during which he rose to play major roles at Blue Cross of Minnesota, went on to inaugurate one of the first HMOs in the country, and later ran HealthPartners in the Twin Cities, a position that prepared Halvorson to run Kaiser Permanente (like Kaiser, HealthPartners owns and operates its own hospitals and has a close affiliation with its doctors). Thirty years of experience prepared Halvorson to ascend to the position as chairman and CEO, Kaiser Foundation Health Plan and Kaiser Foundation Hospitals, the largest nonprofit health plan in the United States with nearly 9 million members, thirty-five hospitals in nine states and the District of Columbia, 13,000 doctors in more than 430 medical offices, and 156,000 employees. CEOs holding such lofty positions don't generally volunteer anecdotes that make them look like country bumpkins, but Halvorson is a man at ease with himself and he seems to enjoy telling the story, perhaps as a way of keeping him tethered to the sturdy Minnesota roots that have served him so well.

Kaiser is a special place. It was born out of necessity during the Great Depression when a visionary young doctor began treating construction workers in the southwestern United States. Employees paid five cents a day for coverage, and the new entity became a combined insurance plan and hospital/physician care delivery system. Thus was born the concept of prepaid, preventive health care.

George Halvorson sports a full beard, struggles with his weight, and has the rumpled air of an academic. His writer's instinctive intellectual curiosity has never waned. Books and ideas matter to him.

He is a corporate chieftain who has studied Darwin, Edward O. Wilson, and James Joyce. Even as he has worked as the leader of major health care companies, he has still carved out time to write, producing four books overall, three in just a four-year span from 2003–2007. His latest, *Health Care Reform Now! A Prescription for Change,* is a relentless indictment of the "current nonsystem of care [as] inconsistent, massively expensive, sometimes dangerous, operationally inefficient, and dysfunctionally and sometimes perversely incented." An earlier book, *Strong Medicine: What's Wrong with America's Health Care System and How We Can Fix It,* was described by Warren Buffett as "by far the clearest explanation of how we have gotten to where we are in health care." An indication of his intellectual range is that he is currently working on a book about racial and ethnic prejudice (a project he's been struggling with since 1987).

Halvorson's knowledge and passion for these issues have made him one of the prominent players in the new quality movement. Among his first acts at Kaiser, in fact, was to hire Louise Liang, MD, as head of quality for the Kaiser system. Dr. Liang had been a colleague of Don Berwick's decades earlier at the Harvard Community Health Plan; she also was a key player at IHI as a board member and, for a time, board chair as well. Halvorson and Liang built a partnership with Berwick and IHI that enables Kaiser personnel and others to learn from various IHI faculty and events. Halvorson and Liang have dispatched Kaiser teams to Jönköping to learn from Göran Henriks and his colleagues, and a Jönköping delegation has visited Kaiser, as well.

Halvorson's work to improve quality in health care goes back thirty-plus years and has included some highly unconventional approaches. While leading HealthPartners in Minnesota, he traveled extensively advising various governments around the world on health policy, including those in Russia and the United Kingdom, and using his expertise to help start health plans in Spain, Jamaica, Uganda, and Nigeria. These activities have become a passion for Halvorson, and he does not engage in them from a distance. He has traveled a good deal through Uganda, and when he learned that poor villages there had active dairy cooperatives he saw an opening: Why not use precisely the same structure and create a health care cooperative? Thus did Halvorson, working with others, apply the co-op model to health care charging villagers ten cents per member per month, a fee many villagers paid with coffee beans, milk, or tea leaves. In rural Ugandan villages, Halvorson could not resist his ever-present impulse to bring technology to health care and in one particular location, he even hooked a computer system into a generator and built electronic records. Over time, those records revealed that the biggest health care expense was the treatment of malaria. This was a fascinating case because it serves as a kind of microcosm of how data can drive efficiency and quality improvement. The data made it clear that reducing the incidence of malaria would reduce the overall cost of care and simultaneously free up clinicians to spend more time with patients. The solution? Netting for villagers at night at a modest cost resulting in a 50 percent reduction in the incidence of malaria in the village, a healthier population, and significant savings. (Halvorson got so involved in the Uganda project that he published a book about it in 2006: *Health Care Co-ops in Uganda: Effectively Launching Micro Health Groups in African Villages*.) This is the essence of Halvorson's vision for transforming health care in the United States: A data-driven system where measurement guides and propels improvement increasing quality, the health of the population and controlling costs.

Health care in a primitive Ugandan village as a model for the United States? Not exactly, of course, although in the crudest sense the village sketches the broad outlines of the system Halvorson envisions at Kaiser: Technology generating excellent data for meaningful measurement, which, in turn, drives clinical competition and improvement and the application of evidence-based care. Halvorson sees these elements—data, measurement, competition/improvement, and evidence-based care—as the foundation of a new system that is far more efficient, produces a healthier population, and controls costs.

Welcome to George Halvorson's health care revolution.

Halvorson is disturbed by what he sees out upon the vast health care landscape. He observes that 70 percent of the nation's cost of care goes to less than 10 percent of the population, largely patients with one or more of five chronic diseases: diabetes, congestive heart failure, coronary artery disease, asthma, and depression.

He seems doubly disturbed by the lack of data in health care because he views data as the lifeblood of improvement. "Any area of health care that has been measured has been improved," he says. More than anything else, the lack of data is owed to the primitive nature of health care information technology (IT). Those seemingly ubiquitous bulging paper files in doctors' offices cannot be sliced, diced, and analyzed the way computerized information can be. Halvorson is a gentle man who avoids harsh words, but he hates paper records. On a day-to-day care level, says Halvorson, "paper kills." He writes that

> because of the paper medical record we don't have the data necessary to track which providers or care teams have achieved the best results for back surgery, knee surgery, or eye surgery. We don't know which oncology group gives patients the longest survival time from Stage II lung cancer, or who does the best job of treating breast cancer and getting it into remission. . . . How can providers with the worst performance levels improve when they have no sense at all that their below-average performance levels could and should be improved?

The problem is that a clinician has no way of knowing whether he or she is performing near the top or bottom of the pack. Many *think* they know. Many *believe* they are among the best; but, in fact, they have little statistical proof. And *reputation is not measurement*.

The dearth of data and measurement contributes to the second missing ingredient—the lack of evidence-based care. Basing care decisions on scientific evidence seems too rudimentary even to discuss, but that stems from the common misperception that the great majority of American health care today is based on rigorous scientific evidence. In fact, Halvorson says, less than half of the care administered in the United States is based on evidence. The rest is prevailing local practice, habit, intuition, or dependent upon the training of a particular clinician.

Halvorson is deeply involved in the effort to advance the cause of evidence-based care. In 2007, he was invited to join one of the most important Institute of Medicine (IOM) committees ever convened: the IOM Roundtable on Evidence-Based Medicine. The committee's mission is to "transform the way evidence on clinical effectiveness is generated and used to improve health and health care." The committee's goal is that "by the year 2020, 90 percent of clinical decisions will be supported by accurate, timely, and up-to-date clinical information, and will reflect the best available evidence."

Trying to gather, synthesize, and apply data on clinical outcomes from a large patient base by using paper records would be like using an abacus to calculate reentry speed for the space shuttle. Virtually every profession in the modern world relies on information technology to improve work. How is it that banking and engineering, for example, are so many light years ahead of health care in the use of technology for quality improvement?

When the headhunter called inquiring whether George Halvorson was interested in the CEO position at Kaiser Permanente, he did not think twice. "No thank you," he said. He was quite happy where he was; he loved Minnesota and HealthPartners, and he had zero interest in leaving. It was partly that he was a Minnesotan through and through, but more than that he was leading an organization for which he felt great passion. A few months later, however, Halvorson's friend Karen Ignagni, president and CEO of the America's Health Insurance Plans (Halvorson serves on the board), called him and said, "George, you're an idiot." She explained that she had just been talking with someone at Kaiser and had learned that Halvorson had declined to talk with them about the CEO position. "I told her, I love Kaiser but that's not the path I'm on," Halvorson recalled.

But this was crazy. Halvorson had a vision for what health care could become, thought about it all the time, had written books about it—and he wasn't *interested*? And then she said something that was a sort of lightning strike: "George, all of the things you want to do to reform health care, you can do at Kaiser and the world will see them and learn."

Halvorson knew she was right, that Kaiser presented the chance to build a twenty-first-century system of care; the most advanced information technology would generate data for measurement and comparison and thus drive quality improvement. If he should get the position, Halvorson would be taking over one of the great health care companies in the world, and he would be succeeding an icon in American health care, David Lawrence, MD. Lawrence was the man who had defined the American system as in such dire shape that "the chassis is broken," and he had served with Berwick and Leape on the Institute of Medicine committee that had produced the *Chasm* report. But by the time Karen Ignagni called Halvorson, the Kaiser folks were nearing the end of their process and had whittled the prospects to a list of finalists. When they heard from Ignagni that Halvorson was now more open-minded about the position, a Kaiser executive traveled to Minnesota for a visit; that conversation, in turn, led to additional discussions and, finally, to an interview with the Kaiser board.

When Halvorson met with the Kaiser board, he told them what he believed was wrong with American health care. He talked about data and measurement, about evidence-based care, and about his belief that technology could produce the kind of data and measurement that would enable quality improvement as never before. He said he believed that technology and evidence-based care could change the world; he also said that if they saw things that way it might be a good fit, but if they did not, he was perfectly happy where he was.

His first mission when he took over Kaiser was to build a great IT system, and here he was working in largely, though not entirely, uncharted territory. A few hospital systems—Geisinger in Pennsylvania and Intermountain in Utah, for example—had built or were in the process of building impressive technology platforms, though they were vastly smaller systems than Kaiser. Although no private company had ever undertaken such an ambitious IT project, the U.S. government—in the form of the Veterans Administration (VA)—had done so. Halvorson was quite familiar with the VA system and its resulting transformation in quality. He had had numerous conversations with the VA leader, Kenneth Kizer, MD, who took over a VA system rife with incompetence and mismanagement. Kizer based the turnaround in large measure on a universal system of Electronic Medical Records (EMR) throughout the system's more than 150 hospitals, 130 nursing homes, and 800-plus clinics. By 1999, Kizer had installed an EMR system that dramatically improved the ability of physicians to administer quality care. Since records were instantly available, physicians had all the relevant information they might need for a patient. Clinicians found the system heading off numerous medication errors every day. Kizer energized the system when he published performance measures for each facility, thus triggering intense competition among doctors and hospitals. "People competed like hell," Kizer told *US News and World Report*.

Beth McGlynn and a team of RAND researchers found in 2005 that the VA was performing some quality miracles—that "VA patients received about two-thirds of the care recommended by national standards, compared with about half in the national sample." RAND found that patients in the national sample received about 20 percent of the recommended care, but VA patients got 65 percent. The report indicated that that on average prescriptions throughout the country were filled correctly anywhere from 92 to 97 percent of the time, but at the VA it was done correctly 99.997 percent of the time. And the VA had accomplished all this at a cost of $5,000 per patient compared to the national cost in the United States of $6,300 per patient. The turnaround at the VA was a huge story in American health care, and, after the improvements were made, Ken Kizer declared without reservation that "the single most important thing that can be done to improve the quality, safety, and efficiency of health care today is to widely implement Electronic Health Records." Unfortunately, Kizer appeared to have stepped on one too many political toes in Washington and was eventually forced out of his position, a move widely lamented throughout the new quality movement.

Halvorson and his Kaiser team learned a great deal from the folks at the VA. The two organizations, in fact, established a strategic partnership to cooperate on EMR standards. Yet the reality was that in the private sector no one had attempted to create an EMR system on so massive a scale as Kaiser. The VA system served 5.4 million patients, but Halvorson wanted to build a system for nearly twice that number. This would have been exceedingly difficult if Halvorson's computerization proposal had been the first time the Kaiser employees had heard this, but it was actually the third. An effort to build a system in 1997 was halted and the organization was in the midst of a second effort as Halvorson arrived.

Kaiser has a long tradition of technological innovation, having computerized some data as far back as the 1960s and 1970s. The technology ethic remained strong within the company and during the 1990s Kaiser locations throughout the country created a variety of award-winning technological approaches. Three separate Kaiser Electronic Health Record installations—in Ohio, the Northwest region, and Colorado—were recognized at different times as the best in the nation. Kaiser executives recognized that the Colorado location in particular had developed a fine Electronic Medical Record. The Colorado operation, in collaboration with IBM, created a system that was among the most advanced in the country; indeed, it was so advanced that it won a national award for best health care IT system.

This system grew from humble origins. During the 1980s, when Andy Wiesenthal was a Permanente pediatrician in Colorado, he simultaneously served as the region's quality improvement officer. In this position he was acutely aware that his colleagues for the most part knew little about quality improvement but this did not deter him. He took the job seriously and was soon frustrated by the lack of data that he felt was necessary to propel improvement. Wiesenthal decided to take matters into his own hands and, in the quiet of his basement, he set about writing software for an Electronic Medical Record. Though he was well educated and possessed epidemiological experience at the Centers for Disease Control, Wiesenthal had no engineering experience and he soon realized he had neither the training or experience to undertake such a task. Eventually, he and his colleagues found their way to IBM, where they teamed up with engineers there in 1991; six years later, he and his IBM associates had created a custom Electronic Medical Record for Kaiser's Colorado region—a record that proved reliable, and popular with clinicians—quite an achievement. While the Colorado system only covered the outpatient medical record it was nonetheless a good start. In 2000, two years before George Halvorson took over at Kaiser, Wiesenthal's success brought him a new assignment: to morph his Colorado system into a national Kaiser system. The project encountered a series of difficult challenges—technical for the most part—yet Wiesenthal persevered; two years later, Kaiser deployed the system at operations in Hawaii and they were literally a matter of weeks away from doing the same in California.

But then George Halvorson arrived.

In the months before he took over at Kaiser, Halvorson talked informally with former and current Kaiser executives and IT consultants, and it became increasingly clear to him that the system was several years out of date—easy to happen in the IT world where the pace of change was so rapid. Halvorson saw the existing system as "a valiant effort that had flaws."

When it came to technology, Halvorson knew what he did not know. He tended to be a pretty self-effacing individual and he did not hide the fact that he had made a technology mistake at Health-Partners, which was originally on a Macintosh system. "I like Apple and really wanted to stick with the Macs, even though my IT department was telling me we needed to switch to PCs," he told a newspaper reporter. "I probably held onto those Macs two years longer than I should have and we ended up playing catch-up with the competition for a few years afterward."

He was not about to make another technology mistake at Kaiser; soon after taking over, he announced a series of changes. He wasn't altogether sure what else was out there in the technical landscape, but he wanted to make sure they turned over every rock in the marketplace before making a final decision. He announced that he was suspending the rollout of the Colorado-IBM system and forming a task force to study the latest technology developments in health care.

When Wiesenthal got wind of the change in technology direction, he was incredulous. Kaiser had already rolled out the system in Hawaii and they were about to do the same in Southern California (making this technology iteration further along than any previous effort) when out of the blue the whole project was put on hold. Wiesenthal was livid. "Here's this guy brand new to the organization," says Wiesenthal, "and we had been working really hard just starting to achieve some success and . . ." Fuming, Wiesenthal followed his usual custom when needing to blow off steam—he went out for a long run. "I was very angry, but the run was very therapeutic," he recalls. And after an hour of running through his anger, dripping with sweat there in Oakland, Andy Wiesenthal came to a realization: *Halvorson was right*.

"He was a brand new CEO and he had every right to take a fresh look at it and see if we were on the right path," says Wiesenthal. "I realized that if I were coming in . . . I'd be doing exactly the same thing. George is a smart guy and he . . . looked at what we were doing and . . . viewed it as sort of typical. He said, 'Look I know a lot of time and money and effort has gone into this, but I think it might be a mistake and I want you to reassess what you've done.'"

Halvorson then asked Wiesenthal and Louise Liang, MD, to lead a task force to go out into the marketplace and find the best possible system for Kaiser. Wiesenthal partnered with Liang, who had been one of Halvorson's first hires upon arriving at Kaiser. She played a central role in the Halvorson-led quality movement at Kaiser. When she and Halvorson arrived Kaiser had no centralized function for measuring quality. Data generated throughout the system was on different IT platforms with differing definitions. Thus, much of the data was not comparable. This was a huge problem because comparable, system-wide data was central to the quality improvement Halvorson and Liang were driving. To improve quality,

Kaiser needed a sturdy platform of data that could only be generated by a uniform Electronic Health Record. Part of Liang's mission was to redesign the system's quality processes to enable collaborative efforts on quality across the system. Liang brought with her professional heft in the form of extensive quality experience, a background working with Berwick at IHI and experience having founded a Permanente medical group. She often said that "Kaiser Permanente is world class in everything, just not everywhere" and it was her mission to change that.

Halvorson knew that Wiesenthal and others had just surveyed the marketplace two and a half years earlier, but he also knew that the technology landscape could change overnight. He was acutely aware that previous studies had shown that a terrifying percentage of health care IT installations—maybe as high as two-thirds—crash and burn. On one level, this was a simple process of selecting a technology platform, but on another level, it was a high-wire act: The reality of this technology search was set against a backdrop of the disastrous experience of another big, prestigious West Coast player—Cedars-Sinai Medical Center in Los Angeles. Cedars had installed an expensive computerized physician order-entry system in 2003 that was intended to improve clinical efficiency and reduce medical errors. Almost immediately after the system was introduced, there were problems. Doctors had difficulty ordering medications. The software seemed difficult to use and, worse, quite time-consuming. Almost overnight doctors grew frustrated. Rumblings, complaints, and frustration grew into a physicians' uprising. Doctors said the system was too complex, inconvenient, hard to use, and imprecise. And then the physicians played their ultimate trump card: *The system as constructed is endangering patient safety.* After just four months in use, under overwhelming pressure from doctors, Cedars shut down the system. What had begun with the best intentions and highest hopes imploded, becoming a cautionary tale for anyone in American health care seeking to use information technology as an important medical tool.

But perhaps the Cedars debacle was a blessing of sorts, an ever-present reminder of how not do it. Halvorson, Liang, and Wiesenthal took an important lesson from the Cedars experience—make sure the doctors drive the bus; make absolutely sure the doctors and other clinicians are essential to the process of selecting the new system.

Andy Wiesenthal and Louise Liang were a strong partnership. Wiesenthal had a background in quality improvement and technology; Liang was a quality movement pioneer, a longtime associate of Berwick's, a mainstay at IHI. She had extensive hospital and medical group experience in changing large systems. In the summer of 2002, their task force scoured the country and quickly found that few companies were capable of handling a project the size and complexity of Kaiser. After an in-depth technical assessment Wiesenthal, Liang, and their team narrowed the possibilities to three: the on-hold internal IBM partnership along with two outside companies: Cerner Corporation of Kansas City and Epic Systems of Madison, Wisconsin.

During the next couple of months, Wiesenthal, Liang, and dozens of members of their task force—along with representatives from all KP regions—fanned out across the country visiting hospitals and physician practices equipped with Cerner and Epic installations. Right from the start, feedback was consistent—quite positive about Epic Systems, not so positive about Cerner. The Kaiser teams would arrive at a hospital or physician practice for a tour in such large numbers that "our vendor shepherds could never really control us," says Wiesenthal. "Whenever we had a tour we had people drift away and talk with their peers—pharmacists slip away and talk with pharmacists, radiologists to radiologists, nurses to nurses, and on and on." These were private conversations, away from the vendor representatives, and they were more revealing than anything. Epic clients liked the system generally and found it fairly easy to use. "With the other vendor people would say, 'This is awful I can't use it' or 'I don't use it I make my resident use it' or 'It's been really problematic and I try to avoid using it,'" recalls Wiesenthal. At the end of the process, the task force was unanimous in its support of Epic.

Halvorson met with leaders of the team, reviewed their thinking, listened to their analysis, and agreed with their recommendation: Epic was the right system. He also knew the ramifications of this—that Kaiser would have to write off the money spent and contractually committed to the Colorado/IBM approach—a staggering $442 *million*. But Halvorson also knew that the Kaiser board was firmly committed to this course and had been from the beginning. The board and Halvorson shared one vision, and they were pursuing it together.

The enormity of the write-down notwithstanding, Halvorson's mission at Kaiser was to create the finest health care technology system anywhere; he wanted to break new ground and provide Kaiser members and physicians with tools that would improve the quality of care by an order of magnitude. He would never waiver from this mission, and in the early days he received some kudos for his efforts. In 2005, Halvorson was one of three winners nationally of the CEO IT Achievement Award sponsored by *Modern Healthcare* and the Healthcare Information and Management Systems Society. One of the judges for the award, a Kansas City hospital president, said of Halvorson: "I was greatly impressed by his leadership in advancing IT on every level—the business level, the clinical level, the patient level—and by his emphasis on measuring and improving quality."

But whatever honeymoon Halvorson might have enjoyed was over by 2006 when controversy and turbulence seemed the rule rather than the exception and he was under intense pressure on various fronts. The California Department of Managed Health Care forced Kaiser to pay $5 million in fines and donations as punishment for delays in its Northern California kidney transplant program, a scandal that left many patients waiting for transplants much longer than necessary.

Halvorson faced a frightening personal issue at home in Minnesota one weekend in April 2006: He was stricken with a serious heart attack and required to undergo bypass surgery. After a few rough months, he was on the road to recovery. But even then, 2006 was not proving to be a particularly pleasant year. In the fall, a young Kaiser employee sent an e-mail around the company criticizing Halvorson and the IT rollout.

As Kaiser went about building the system, Halvorson knew there would be technical issues—and, of course, there were. Some were handled quickly; others were more difficult and required significant expense to repair. During 2006, the system was up and running from 98 percent to 99.7 percent of the time, but it crashed for more than fifty hours from May 9 to May 11 (due to a power outage); during that time, doctors and pharmacists were unable to retrieve critical patient information. The situation proved to be a surprisingly important experience. A major reason so many health care IT installations fail is that doctors never adapt—they just don't use the system and over time it becomes an expensive relic. When the power failed in Corona, California, where Kaiser then had its primary data center and the Kaiser system went down, doctors were furious. They wanted their system back up and running! In a way, this was a great test because it revealed that the doctors were not only using the system but relying upon it.

As though enough unpleasantness hadn't marked the year, a rumor made its way onto the Internet that Halvorson held a personal stake in Epic, the IT vendor the company had chosen, in spite of the fact that Epic was a closely held private concern and Halvorson had no such connection. On top of it all a bogus yet authentic-looking press release reached news outlets in the final weeks of 2006 announcing that Halvorson was resigning immediately. Although a hoax, it nonetheless added to the general air of negativity. Newspaper headlines such as "Kaiser Denies Its Herculean IT Conversion Project in Trouble" didn't help much. The difficulties spilled into 2007 with the release of the Michael Moore film *SICKO*, which attacked Kaiser. The film told of an eighteen-month-old child who died at a Los Angeles Kaiser hospital in 1993 and asserted that Kaiser had denied the child a blood test that might have revealed her condition. Kaiser's response was that the child's death had nothing to do with its policies or practices and that the case was extremely unfortunate malpractice by two non-Kaiser physicians (who were subsequently convicted of malpractice in the case, as was the hospital). The movie also covered a case where a Kaiser hospital sent a sixty-three-year-old homeless patient—dressed in a hospital gown and shoeless—to a Skid Row shelter in Los Angeles. Kaiser officials apologized to the woman and conceded that it had been a horrendous mistake. The incident brought down the Los Angeles county attorney's wrath (as well as attention to violations by other LA County health systems); Kaiser paid a fine and established a specific protocol for the release of homeless patients to insure their safety, a protocol the regional ACLU director characterized as "the most comprehensive, broad-based and sensitive protocol for hospital discharge planning for homeless patients resulting from any case in the nation's history."

Through all the unpleasantness, Halvorson, his leadership team, and the Kaiser board kept their focus. The board, in fact, has been steadfast in its pursuit of quality improvements. Liang and her staff were instrumental in helping create a committee of the board which oversees the organization's quality improvement efforts and established the policies that enabled Liang to redesign the quality process throughout Kaiser, a tedious but meaningful exercise.

From the outset Halvorson made a decision that the company would spend whatever it took to get the system built properly as quickly as possible. Halvorson was unafraid of breaking a budget here or there if it meant getting closer to the goal. He told the board of directors: "We're laying track just in front of the train and the train's rolling right behind and if we get to a river and the bridge isn't there we're going to parachute in enough consultants to build that bridge before the train gets here. We're not going to stop, rethink, re-budget, reallocate because the most important thing we're doing strategically is to put the system in place."

Halvorson is a generally calm man, but he could not help hold his breath at least a bit to wait for feedback on the new system. There were problems and complaints, of course, but these were over-whelmed by the positive feedback from throughout Kaiser installations across the country.

Nobody knew the system—its weaknesses, strengths and potential—better than Andy Wiesenthal, and at the beginning of 2008, when the system was up and running nearly everywhere, he was ec-static. Although some of the transition was difficult, the adoption generally went quite smoothly and the feedback from Kaiser hospitals and physician practices, was largely positive. Says Wiesenthal:

> This fundamentally means that whatever information we have is available twenty-four hours, seven days, 365 days a year. You never ever have to make a clinical decision about a patient without information. I cannot tell you what that means to me as a doctor. You've learned over a lifetime to function in the absence of information—the chart is in a different office or hospital or it's lost or out to somebody else or it's missing. In America we think it's okay to take the sickest people and put them in front of doctors and nurses and give them *nothing* to go on [a reference to emergency room visits]. They don't know anything and they have to make decisions and take care of you. Now that never has to happen again—ever.

Wiesenthal says nurses estimate that in a paper record system they spend about 15 percent of their time each day looking for records, orders, charts—pieces of paper. "Fifteen percent of the day for a trained professional looking for paper," he says, "and now it's zero. You can't imagine how transformative that is."

Wiesenthal and Liang point to how the system is having an immediate and dramatic impact in many areas of safety and quality. With all medications prescribed through the system the chance of a medication error —the most common type of medical mistake—is significantly reduced. In Hawaii, a Kaiser nephrologist used the IT database to identify every diabetic in the region and then targeted every one who had not been screened for potential renal failure. Those members were brought in and screened so effectively that the physician has been able to reduce dramatically the need for dialysis among his patients.

The key element of success was that Kaiser built a clinician-driven system. They had adopted a system the doctors had checked out and liked. This, says Wiesenthal, was in contrast to the Cedars project. "Ours is a physician/clinician–led project. It is *not* an information technology–led project. At Cedars it was led by IT and done *to* the doctors and the doctors didn't like it."

Mark Groshek, a Kaiser pediatrician in Colorado, finds the system easy to use and highly efficient. "As a pediatrician I have growth charts in the system which I show to parents to show how their child is growing: a nice, simple graphic that tells them how things are going." Lab results arrive quickly; no one has to go down to a different floor or make phone calls to get them. A patient instruction section is particularly useful because it enables Groshek to type into a template precisely what the parents should do for home care. Sometimes there are a number of items, and often when those instructions are verbal parents can forget or get confused. With the IT system the instructions print out clearly.

The online personal health record portion of the system has been embraced by both clinicians and patients (and their parents). Parents with sick children send Groshek an e-mail detailing symptoms and asking whether the child should be seen. Quite often, the kids do not need to come into the office, saving the family time and inconvenience and changing the makeup of Groshek's schedule to focus not on how many patients he sees in a day, but to look more broadly at how many patient problems/concerns he can address. The online system is particularly helpful with chronic-disease patients because close monitoring of their various functions is so critical. With asthma patients, for example, parents send Groshek peak flow numbers via e-mail, thus avoiding the need for an office or lab visit but at the same time enabling Groshek to stay abreast of the results.

One of the most important functions of the system is that it enables primary care doctors to consult specialists in any field, secure in the knowledge that they are looking at identical information. A primary care doctor may want to consult a specialist ten miles away, or a hundred miles, or a thousand miles. With the system, he or she can do so; and although the doctors are in separate offices, they are both looking at the same information—the same image—on their computer screens.

"The system gives us all of the information about all of our patients all of the time," says Halvorson. "The doctor who's treating the patient knows everything there is to know about that patient. They know what prescriptions they're on, what tests they've had, what their track record has been so the doctor can make better, more informed decisions about the patient—far better than they can make with a subset of data."

The Kaiser system includes best-practice alerts that guide doctors on medications and treatments. Built into the foundation of the system are evidence-based guidelines that the clinician can rely upon in real time in the exam room. The clinical best-practice guidelines are not pulled from thin air. Kaiser has built an internal unit—the Care Management Institute—that "synthesizes knowledge on the best clinical approaches from both within and outside Kaiser Permanente, then develops integrated care management programs." The professionals at the institute scour major sources of best-practice guidelines—professional societies, medical journals—and integrate that information with internal ongoing research at Kaiser. The result is a seamless flow of the very latest information on a variety of clinical topics through the Kaiser IT system to doctors, nurses, and technicians. Clinicians are able to access the information anywhere and at any time. The institute's focus is currently on the five major chronic diseases—asthma, coronary artery disease, depression, diabetes and heart failure—as well as cancer, chronic pain, and elder care.

Along with measurement, the system's decision-support function is key to improving quality, says Halvorson. He notes that a generation ago only a few hundred medical journal articles annually provided new best-practice treatments; today, there are more than 30,000 each year, and no doctor has the capability to recall a fraction of those while sitting in an exam room with a patient. But the computer does it with ease.

While working on a book with George Isham, MD, of Health-Partners, Halvorson "looked at 135 doctors who were asked how they would treat a particular condition for a particular patient. They came up with eighty-two separate treatments. Why? Because some physicians graduated from medical school last month. Others graduated a year ago, or twenty years ago, or forty years ago. Some attended seminars on the topic. Others read articles on the topic. Some articles were recent. Some weren't." The decision-support function offers a solution to this problem by providing best-practice recommendations to doctors and nurses in real time at the point of care. While Kaiser is embarked upon among the most ambitious IT journeys in the country, there are other health care organizations moving in a similar direction. Intermountain in Utah, for example, was a pioneer with Electronic Medical Records as far back as the mid-1990s when Brent James, MD, and his colleagues began using records to improve clinical care and to gather improvement data. James and his colleagues are now building a new system in partnership with General Electric (GE). They looked at the major vendors—Epic and Cerner included—and concluded that at Intermountain, working in collaboration with GE, they could create something more flexible and responsive to their own needs. James expects the system to be up and running in 2010.

The Geisinger Health System in northeastern and central Pennsylvania has constructed one of the most advanced systems anywhere. With 700 physicians spread across forty sites covering 20,000 square miles, the Geisinger doctors long ago recognized the need for computerized records that could be easily shared. In the mid–1990s, Geisinger initiated an effort to build an EMR system that was up and running across most of the system by 2003 (Geisinger contracts with Epic and was one of the sites the Kaiser team visited before selecting Epic as their vendor). Today, that system is a model for what many others hope to accomplish and while it is a fraction of the size of the Kaiser system, it is similarly ambitious in its effort to improve quality.

Ronald Paulus, MD, chief health information technology venture officer, notes that Geisinger's EMR system provides the tools for significant improvement. With diabetes, for example, the Geisinger team identified nine specific steps that all diabetics should take each year to keep their disease under control. The IT system tells Paulus precisely where every patient stands in terms of compliance with the nine items. Further, when a patient makes an appointment to see a physician, the computer screen shows what tests are needed and automatically alerts personnel to schedule the tests for when the patient is there. The system lists all nine items on one screen, thus enabling a nurse or a doctor to see in seconds precisely where a patient stands. The entire system is based upon the idea of applying evidence-based care to drive measurable improvement in quality.

The computer system generates results for each physician and each physician group. Every doctor—and every group—is able to see where he or she stands compared to peers and how each group stands compared to the average and the best. When the comparisons were first published, there was something of a culture shock. When results for a group of measures comprising the diabetes bundle were released, many doctors were taken aback and challenged the accuracy of the data. As Paulus recalls: "People said, 'The numbers can't possibly be true.'" But over time doctors have come to accept their accuracy; indeed, individuals and groups not near the top have made vigorous competitive efforts to improve. "Once they got past the fact that the numbers were right, people were highly energized to make it better," says Paulus. "The entire dialogue shifted to 'Let's go, let's make it better.'"

And they have done just that. From March 2006 to December 2007, the Geisinger team made measurable progress on the nine metrics of care identified as best practice. Influenza vaccination went from 57 percent of patients in March 2006 to 71 percent in December 2007; pneumococcal vaccination went from 57 percent to 71 percent, and microalbumin order from 58 percent to 88 percent. Similar improvements were apparent in the bundle of services for coronary artery disease.

Like Geisinger and others, the Kaiser system includes health reminder alerts so that when a patient comes in for a visit the computer signals whether the patient is due for tests or screenings. In one instance in 2006, a woman went to a Kaiser facility in Southern California. She told her story in a brief letter to the physician in charge of the medical center:

Early last year, I came to your facility to have a foreign body removed from my eye. I visited your Ophthalmology Department and your competent staff dealt with this minor emergency. What made this visit so meaningful was my interaction with your nurse after my visit with the doctor. In addition to giving me some after-visit instructions, she noticed in the computer that I needed a mammography exam. I had been reminded before but I tend to be too busy to take care of my own health. This time the nurse was very insistent. She even made me an appointment so I could walk in and get the exam within the hour.

Since I did not have to wait too long, I had the exam done that day. Well, they found a mass in my right breast and it was cancer. I have gone through chemotherapy and radiation therapy and today I am cancer free.

I am convinced that I am alive today because of your organization's focus on my total health. My interaction with your entire health care system has been nothing but positive. I am especially appreciative to the young nurse who took the time to convince a stubborn old lady to take responsibility for my health. Thank you for giving me many more years to thrive.

The essential ambition at Kaiser was to use the best technology to transform primary care delivery: to enable front-line clinicians such as Dr. Groshek to provide the highest possible quality of care. Patients also play a critical role in home care and are assisted by personal health records that connect them electronically to their doctors, nurses, and pharmacists. The use of these personal health records has enabled patients to help manage their own care more efficiently and has directly resulted in fewer office visits and phone calls to clinicians. Patients know the results of lab tests as soon as they are posted. They can double or triple check the physician's directions concerning pharmaceuticals by going online. If a patient is confused, he or she can easily fire off an e-mail message to the doctor, nurse, or pharmacist.

With the aging of the baby boom generation, an increasing number of families include elderly parents who are helped or cared for by their adult children. With permission, the adult children gain access to their parents' health records to check medications, understand proposed treatments, and query clinicians. When confused, an elderly parent calls an adult child who, in turn, goes online and finds the information in the parent's record.

From a patient's standpoint, it's not just about computers. Halvorson envisions a day in the not-too-distant future when people use their everyday communications tools in health care. A huge percentage of the Kaiser members, for example have cell phones—many more than have computers. Much of the communication now done by computers will be achievable by cell phones in just a few years. An essential element of quality care, in fact, stems from good communications. Patients at home, particularly those suffering from chronic illnesses, will be able to transmit data concerning their weight, blood sugar levels, blood pressure, and so forth, through their mobile devices—laptop, PDA, or cell phone.

Halvorson ruminates on what he considers a fundamental flaw in American health care: improperly aligned financial incentives. "As a pure business model, health care is winning," he says. "Health care is taking all . . . your money and is doing it without having to be particularly accountable in how the money's spent. Based on that, health care will never, ever reform itself. The model is too lucrative." He likes to point out that there are something like 10,000 billing codes in health care for procedures, but as he told *Healthcare Today*: "There are no billing codes for cures. There are no billing codes for outcomes. There are no billing codes for care improvement." If the focus is on the volume of procedures, then it is volume we get, more volume than anywhere else on the planet, he says. "Providers," he adds, "don't do what they're not paid to do."

That is why he thinks the Kaiser model makes so much sense as a way to combat the inherent problems in health care today. Kaiser's structure is not unique, but it is different from most. In most places throughout the United States there are three major separate health care players: Hospitals, doctor's groups, and insurance companies. With Kaiser, it's all effectively under one roof—and that makes a huge difference in what Kaiser has the incentive to do. Kaiser is paid a certain amount to care for a population of patients. The healthier Kaiser can keep those patients, the more money Kaiser makes (though it is a nonprofit, the funds are essential to the company's financial health and ability to fulfill its mission). Thus, the member wins, as does Kaiser.

Take diabetes, for example. At Kaiser, a program to treat every diabetes patient with evidence-based care and thus keep them out of the hospital yields to Kaiser's financial benefit—since Kaiser's greatest cost is when patients are admitted to its hospitals. In a typical arrangement, however, a hospital that cares for a diabetic population so well that it eliminates hospital admissions is doing financial harm to itself—a powerful disincentive. In essence, the healthier Kaiser can keep a patient the more money it saves for its members. In most hospitals, the sicker a patient the more the hospital makes—which is why so many health plans and hospitals throughout the country are experimenting with contracts that pay hospitals for keeping patients healthy rather than for procedures. It also explains the trend toward the increased use of Electronic Medical Records; only with a powerful IT system can hospitals and physician groups actually measure quality of care, and if they are eventually going to be paid for quality rather than for procedures they need the ability to measure outcomes.

In 2005, Halvorson predicted that by 2010 people will look back at how doctors practiced that year and view it as "a kind of medical

Dark Ages." He is convinced that the case for constructing systems of Electronic Health Records is so overwhelming that it will soon be the rule rather than the exception. In December 2007, with the Kaiser system up and running, a *Wall Street Journal* survey by Harris Interactive found that American adults strongly believe in the efficacy of Electronic Medical Records. The survey reported that "74 percent believe that patients could receive better care if doctors and researchers were able to share information more easily via electronic medical systems; 63 percent believe that the use of Electronic Medical Records could significantly decrease the frequency of medical errors, and 60 percent believe that the benefits of Electronic Medical Records outweigh the privacy risks." A study published in the summer of 2007 by the Integrated Healthcare Association, a California quality improvement group, showed that California physician groups using IT scored significantly better on a range of clinical measures than their counterparts not using IT.

Halvorson has a perfect-storm theory. He believes that circumstances and events are aligning to propel the new quality movement to the tipping point. He contends that the major players have grown acutely aware of the problem and are impatient with the lack of solutions, and he sees a growing conviction among the buyers of care, government policymakers, and leaders in business and academia that the system is deeply flawed. Until now, he says, there has been no grassroots uprising and thus no broad-based push for improvement. But so many stakeholders are calling for change that he believes the pace of it will accelerate. He sees the educational and research work done in recent years by key players in the movement—the IOM, Berwick and IHI, RAND and, more recently, the Commonwealth Fund—as building to a critical mass.

He thinks the revolution has come.

11

The Holy Grail

———⊶⊷———

"They think I'm a dreamer."

Don Berwick watched as dozens, then hundreds, and finally thousands of doctors, nurses, technicians, medical students, academics, hospital CEOs and trustees—more than 6,000 strong—surged into the Marriott World Center Convention complex in Orlando for the 2007 IHI Forum. In the early morning, as people arrived in buses, rental cars, taxis, and vans, the sun shone brightly and the temperature climbed toward its high of eighty-two degrees for the day. The participants had come from all fifty states, every continent, and thirty-five foreign nations—from Romania and Thailand, Singapore and South Africa, Argentina and Norway—some arriving after twenty-four hours of continuous travel. Since the 2,000 rooms at the Marriott itself had been snapped up eight months earlier, several thousand delegates booked into another dozen-plus hotels scattered throughout the Greater Orlando area. Thousands had been to previous IHI Forums—many to a half dozen or more. This year, the new quality movement's growth was reflected in the fact that more than half the attendees (3,712 out of 6,235) were there for the first time.

As Berwick worked his way through the massive convention center greeting old friends and colleagues with whom he'd fought the good fight for thirty years, he beamed as he spotted some and embraced others, all the while meeting new converts from throughout the world. Don Berwick wore gray slacks and a tweed jacket with a blue button-down shirt and conservative tie. Most of the participants were dressed more casually, the vast majority of men tie-less, but for Berwick this was IHI's grandest event of the year. Everywhere Berwick looked he saw someone who reminded him of progress on some aspect of quality. There was Gary Kaplan from Virginia Mason, Uma Kotagal and Jim Anderson from Cincinnati Children's, a team from Kaiser Permanente, and a delegation a dozen strong from Jönköping, Sweden. And, of course, there was Sorrel King, an eternal reminder for Berwick of why he must get up each and every day and fight as hard as he possibly can.

There was something inspiring about it all, delegates forsaking the tennis courts and lush golf course for hard work over the course of four days. In all, there were 178 class offerings taught by an experienced faculty. Classroom subjects included *Driving Towards Zero: Preventing Health Care Associated Infections; Using Better Real Time Data to Monitor Improvement; Keys to Sustaining Improvement; Door to Balloon Time in Acute Myocardial Infarction; Leading Large-Scale Change and the Role of the CEO.* There were classes on the use of IT, on the Baldrige National Quality Program, on the next generation of pay for performance, on family-centered care, on hand hygiene, and scores more. During the four days, the participants sequestered themselves in the air-chilled convention complex, ducking out into the sunshine at lunch for twenty minutes of warmth and rays. Otherwise they worked, they studied, they taught, they learned, they networked, always searching for ideas to take home and apply at the bedside as soon as possible.

Watching Berwick chat with doctors and nurses, listening intently as some told him of new ideas from their hospitals, it was hard not to recall the early days back at the Harvard Community Health Plan when he had struggled so mightily to find his way on quality. It was impossible not to recall that infamous scene in which Berwick's studious report was balled up and tossed at him.

How far he had traveled since that day! Meeting Paul Batalden and Deming, visits with NASA and Bell Labs, NDP and the HCA courses, the Birthday Club and the birth of IHI, Lucian Leape's error work, *To Err* and *Chasm*, a knighthood, countless awards, scores of articles and books, and hundreds and hundreds of speeches. Such a remarkably rich history! The buzzing energy of the Forum and the sheer passion and brainpower devoted to quality improvement were deeply affirming for Berwick and stood in stark contrast to the time when Berwick, Paul Batalden, and the others had gathered together as the Birthday Club—meeting in airport conference rooms in Chicago and Nashville and Boston and talking about ideas and ambitions that would have sounded heretical or foolish to many at the time. But at the Marriott World Center, ideas derived from those thoughts and ambitions were the mainstream thinking of the new quality movement. The visionaries who had created this movement were seeing a new and immensely rewarding reality.

During this uplifting period, Berwick added to his collection of awards, winning one for being "a catalyst for change" and leading IHI as "a major incubator of innovative concepts"; winning another as "an effective advocate for implementing evidence-based interventions and system strategies designed to protect patients from harm and save lives." He also won the "Purpose Prize" (which carries a $100,000 grant and is awarded to people older than sixty for important contributions to society) largely for the work of the IHI *100,000 Lives* and 5 *Million Lives* campaigns. Perhaps the most telling honor Berwick received during that period, however, came in 2006 when *Modern Healthcare* ranked him as the third most powerful person in American health care (behind the U.S. health and human services secretary and Bill Gates—and one slot ahead of the president). This was the second time Berwick had been so honored. In 2002—largely on the strength of his roles in the two major IOM reports—*Modern Healthcare* placed Berwick third on the list behind the secretary of health and human services and the administrator of the Centers for Medicare and Medicaid Services. In October 2006, an article in *Modern Healthcare* paid Berwick the ultimate compliment by comparing him with perhaps the most important figure in the early history of the quality movement—Ernest Codman, a Boston doctor who pioneered quality a century ago.

There were still skeptics, though their numbers were shrinking. Just over a year before the 2007 Forum, an editor involved with the *US News* "Best American Hospitals" rankings asked Berwick what hospital CEOs and trustees really thought of him. The implication, of course, was that CEOs and trustees constituted the essential health care establishment and that Berwick was the barbarian at the gate. It was a very good question, in fact, for it was a clever way to measure the level of acceptance of the new quality movement in executive suites and boardrooms. Berwick must have been in one of his not so optimistic periods at the time because his answer was this: "No one calls me up and says, 'You're a jerk.' In my heart, I think most of them think I'm unrealistic and don't understand the true world of management of institutions and organizations in a very hostile economic and political climate. They think I am a dreamer."

And, of course, he was. He was a physician, a policy analyst, a research scientist, an orator, a writer, and a leader. And, yes, without question, he was a dreamer.

Berwick himself was not immune from criticism. Early in 2007, David Burda, the editor of *Modern Healthcare,* wrote a somewhat whimsical piece that focused on, of all people, Berwick and Newt Gingrich. Burda characterized both men as sacred cows and then launched into an entertaining and provocative characterization of them as reminiscent of characters from the movie *Animal House.* Berwick was the suave, persuasive fraternity leader—the character called "Otter"—and Gingrich was the unforgettable John Belushi character "Bluto." Even as he was criticizing Berwick, Burda characterized him as "the charismatic leader of the patient-safety movement" able to "pressure even the biggest skeptics into going along with the cause." (Burda was referring to the decision of the American Hospital Association (AHA) to join the IHI 5 *Million Lives* campaign after choosing not to participate in the *100,000 Lives* effort.) "Who dares question Berwick or his actions?" Burda asked, adding that anyone who did so would be "stoned as a heretic." Burda wondered whether the AHA had joined because of Berwick's persuasiveness and the fear of possible bad public relations if it failed to participate. The article was interesting on several counts—Berwick generally enjoyed a favorable press (and was frequently referred to in *Modern Healthcare* in fact as a "guru"). And Berwick was generally viewed as a man of substance, but Burda was suggesting that perhaps Berwick was using his PR savvy to twist the AHA's arm. (Berwick surely stands as the only person ever to be compared—in the same publication no less—to both the legendary Dr. Ernest Codman and the iconic "Otter" of *Animal House,* a rare and enduring distinction.)

Just as the year or so leading up to the 2007 IHI Forum had been a productive period for Berwick, so, too, had it been a robust time for IHI and the quality movement overall. Despite some low moments when Berwick was frustrated by the lack of progress, the movement surged forward during 2006 and 2007, growing broader and deeper and gaining new ground in the mainstream of American health care. For years, the movement's essential battle had been about awareness. For years, too few stakeholders had recognized the quality problem, but by the 2006/2007 period that long and hard-fought battle had been won. Nobody, it seemed, was unaware any longer. "It's no secret anymore we have serious gaps in quality," Berwick said shortly after the conference concluded. "There's much more awareness and much more preparedness for action." Histori-cally, among the least aware health care stakeholders had been trustees on hospital boards, but at the 2007 Forum Berwick saw a number of hospital boards arrive en masse and get right to work. They booked workrooms where, between Forum sessions, they met as a board to work on quality improvement. The notion of hospital trustees becoming "stewards of change," as Berwick put it, was a crucial step forward.

And then there was the breakthrough *100,000 Lives* campaign, a life-saving effort to apply best practices in crucial areas of care. More than 3,000 hospitals participated and the campaign won the active support of the broad medical establishment in the United States— truly a landmark moment in the new quality movement history. The campaign had originated with a conversation Berwick had with his son, Dan, who was working as a political organizer. Don Berwick found Dan's ability to focus on a specific date—a defined end-point— as attractive. Don was feeling at the time that the quality movement was endless, and the idea of setting specific dates for achievements was appealing. During the discussion, Dan said something that res-onated with his father: "Some is not a number, soon is not a time."

This generated Don's idea to set a date—June 14, 2006—to achieve the specific goal of preventing the deaths of the 100,000 U.S. hospital patients the IOM had estimated die from prevent-able medical errors each year. The campaign commenced in Janu-ary 2005 and immediately, Berwick knew it was something special. He reached out to a variety of regulatory and professional groups—including the American Medical Association, the Centers for Medicare & Medicaid Services, the Joint Commission, the American Nurses Association—and invited them to participate. These were central members of the medical establishment, and Berwick was not at all certain what the reaction would be for this was a case where the IHI was moving into front-line clinical care with clearly prescribed methods of treatment. It was possible that the AMA or any other group could have told him to back off, but the response was the opposite: Virtually every group Berwick asked embraced the campaign. Hundreds of places had innovated to improve quality and safety, and the time had come to "harness those experiences and apply the best methods reliably 100 percent of the time." The campaign's life-saving prescription involved six specific steps:

1. Create rapid response teams and deploy them "at the first sign of patient decline."
2. Deliver reliable, evidence-based care for acute myocardial infarction to prevent deaths from heart attack.
3. Prevent adverse drug events by implementing medication reconciliation.
4. Prevent central line infections by implementing a series of interdependent, scientifically grounded steps called the "Central Line Bundle."
5. Prevent surgical site infections by reliably delivering the correct perioperative antibiotics at the proper time.
6. Prevent ventilator-associated pneumonia by implementing a series of interdependent, scientifically grounded steps.

The fundamental belief of the campaign was that these steps would significantly reduce morbidity and mortality. The IHI recognized that the appetites for the campaign menu would vary widely with some hospitals ready to tackle it all and others struggling to take on one of the items. All were welcomed into the program, and the result was that 3,000 hospitals throughout the country signed up. "We struck oil," says Berwick. "The amount of resonance, will, energy level, graciousness, and enrollees—they're an order of magnitude higher than I ever expected."

There were critics of the campaign who argued that IHI had overstated the effectiveness of *100,000 Lives*, but even an author critical of the numbers noted that "that's not saying the campaign did not save lives or was not the right thing to do. We believe it was." IHI, with a rough calculation, figured that well in excess of 100,000 lives were saved by participating hospitals implementing campaign plans and other innovations.

IHI followed with the 5 *Million Lives* campaign intended to protect 5 million patients from preventable medical errors over a two-year period (concluding in December 2008). The new campaign asked hospitals to implement the six strategies from the *100,000 Lives* campaign in addition to six new ones: preventing harm from medications, reducing surgical complications, preventing pressure ulcers, reducing methicillin-resistant *Staphylococcus aureus* (MRSA) infections, delivering "evidence-based care for congestive heart failure to avoid readmissions," and getting hospital trustees to accelerate quality work. In launching the campaign, IHI estimated that approximately "15 million instances of medical harm occur in the U.S. each year—a rate of over 40,000 per day."

The new campaign got underway with 3,700 hospitals signed on (of the approximately 5,700 hospitals in the country), 600-plus more than the previous campaign. In the fall of 2007, ten months into the campaign, IHI conducted what it called a "harvest" of ideas and information by dispatching IHI faculty and staff members to hundreds of hospitals in all fifty states to gather "ideas, innovations, and best practices." The IHI crews logged 275,000 air miles during a two-week "harvesting" period and returned to Cambridge laden with fresh insights. Notably, a few of their key beliefs were reinforced. Improvement was all about leadership; with the Rick Shannons, the Gary Kaplans, and the Uma Kotagals of the world, improvement happens because the leadership is so clear, strong, and directed. Transparency is key. Data that tracks performance drives improvement. There were other lessons, of course, but these were clearly the foundational elements of improvement. Berwick calls the two campaigns "the biggest surprise of my career." Instead of resistance, there was broad support from the medical establishment. Doctors and nurses working on the front lines impressed Berwick with their strength of will to improve and their sheer joyfulness upon seeing evidence of improvement. In an industry where changes in clinical practice could take years or even decades, the progress made in just eighteen months was remarkable.

By 2008, the national conversation about health care had changed. Although much of it still centered on access and cost, now quality and safety were headline issues as well. Paul Batalden believes a "tapestry of threads" explains the progress. Rather than the work of any particular group or individual, Batalden sees a convergence of many forces, including professional development groups and regulatory and accrediting bodies.

During the early years of the twenty-first century, the quality movement was in part fueled by an increased body of work that challenged bedrock notions about American health care, and the granite in the bedrock was the solemn belief that American health care was the best in the world. This was an article of faith, a mantra. But it was no longer unquestioned. And at the core of this sustained reality check was RAND, of course, with work from Bob Brook, Beth McGlynn, and colleagues. But the new kid on the research block was the Commonwealth Fund, a New York–based foundation that generates a steady stream of information and analysis, much of it comparing the performance of U.S. states to one another, but much also comparing the United States on various metrics against the rest of the world.

The Commonwealth Fund's body of work in recent years has challenged the essential conceit in America that contends we have the finest health care system anywhere. In study after study, the group has shown that the United States falls behind in quality, safety, and efficiency. The inescapable conclusion is that although we are spending double or more per capita on health care than any other industrialized nation, we are not getting any better results; indeed, in many cases our results are worse, the vast spending gap notwithstanding. A study supported by the Commonwealth Fund, for example, compared preventable deaths in nineteen industrialized nations and found that the United States ranked last. *Measuring the Health of Nations: Updating an Earlier Analysis*, published in *Health Affairs*, found that fourteen Western European nations along with Australia, Canada, Japan, and New Zealand, did a better job of providing the kind of timely and effective care that prevented mortality in patients younger than seventy-five. The authors indicated that if the United States had merely achieved the average rating of the nations in the study, it would have seen 101,000 fewer deaths each year. Additionally sobering comparative statistics from the Commonwealth Fund indicate that the United States ranks thirty-first in life expectancy and thirty-sixth in infant mortality.

In addition to its research and analysis work, the Commonwealth Fund is reaching for the stars with its Commission on a High Performance Health System, whose goal is to design a system that provides universal access to care that is safe, efficient, and high quality. The commission is promoting transparency, financial incentives for quality and the expansion of electronic health records. (The commission, chaired by James J. Mongan, MD, president and CEO of Partners Healthcare System, includes among its members Maureen Bisognano, George Halvorson, and Cleve Killingsworth.)

The sustained—or, perhaps, relentless—statistical and analytical reality check the Commonwealth Fund provides helped awaken U.S. health care stakeholders. Debunking essential beliefs—articles of faith—is not easy; but, slowly and steadily, research from the Commonwealth Fund and other sources is eroding the sense of self-assurance and deflating some of the arrogance inherent in American health care. Perhaps, most important, it fuels the competitive fires of clinicians who cannot settle for being anything but the best, driving them toward ever greater quality improvement efforts.

Working along a slightly different track was another influential organization: the Joint Commission. When the IHI Forum opened in December 2007, it had been nearly twenty years since the Birth-day Club members, including Jim Roberts, MD, of the commis-sion, had convened to talk about how to get the commission more involved in the movement. During the intervening years, thanks in no small part to Jim Roberts's work, as well as the visionary leader-ship of former Joint Commission CEO Dennis O'Leary, MD, the commission had become a powerful force for quality improvement in hospitals throughout the country. In its annual report on quality and safety for 2007, the Joint Commission found that although there was still a long way to go, American hospitals "continue to show measurable improvements in health care quality and patient safety" and that "patients are more consistently receiving these . . . 'evidence-based' treatments." The commission's focus on quality improvement "legitimized overnight a concern about improvement in every place accredited by the Joint Commission," observes Paul Batalden.

And it was not just the Commonwealth Fund and the Joint Com-mission, of course. Other major regulatory and professional bodies—and even private foundations—played significant roles in advancing the movement as well, including the National Quality Forum; the Hospital Quality Alliance; the Leapfrog Group; the National Patient

Safety Foundation; and the Robert Wood Johnson Foundation, which had long been a pioneer in the quality movement.

So what *is* the state of the new quality movement? Where does it stand today and what lies ahead? Berwick sees two separate yet parallel tracks, and he is as buoyed by progress in one area as he is chagrined by lack of it in another. One of the parallel lines—the inside track—runs through hospitals and physician practices, and here Berwick is energized. The outside track travels through a broad sphere of financing, incentives, and structure, and here Berwick is deeply concerned.

First, the good news on the inside track. "The likelihood that hospital-based acute care safety and reliability will continue to improve is very strong," observes Berwick. He sees large numbers of skilled, committed clinicians and countless successes in quality improvement projects—and, in fact, thousands of the people working on those projects are gathered together in Orlando. "We will likely see a pretty substantial shift in the quality of inpatient care in a substantial number of places. I'm optimistic about that."

It is important not to overstate the case, of course, for there remain too many outposts that have not gotten the message. Consider Rhode Island Hospital in Providence, where three wrong-site surgeries occurred in 2007 alone, with the third coming a matter of weeks before the IHI Forum. The latest involved drilling into the wrong side of the patient's skull.

Rhode Island Hospital aside, scores of hospitals throughout the country are doing good work. A large group of hospitals in Minnesota, for example, got together and decided not to charge patients for a list of twenty-seven so-called "never events"—mistakes such as patient falls that cause harm, leaving a foreign body inside the patient, transfusion of incompatible blood, wrong-site surgeries, and so forth. The Massachusetts Hospital Association pursued a similar course. In Michigan, hospitals got together and shared best-practice information on preventing infections and soon had the lowest infection rate of any state in the country. Improvement work is flourishing throughout the country, from Intermountain in Salt Lake City to McLeod in Greenville, South Carolina; from Geisinger Health System in Danville, Pennsylvania, to Dartmouth in Hanover, New Hampshire; from Cleveland Clinic to Beth Israel Deaconess Medical Center in Boston.

One of the key contributors to advance the movement was the Centers for Medicare & Medicaid Services (CMS), generally viewed as the most powerful health care organization in the United States. A few months before the 2007 IHI Forum, CMS announced a milestone: Medicare was refusing to pay for the treatment of preventable medical errors. Medicare's message to hospitals and physicians throughout the country was: *Enough is enough*—we will not pay for treating "conditions that could reasonably have been prevented," such as certain hospital-acquired infections, pressure ulcers, injuries sustained in falls within the hospital, and surgical-site infections after coronary artery bypass surgery. Until Medicare took its stand, health plans routinely spent millions of dollars, perhaps billions, to pay hospitals to heal patients they had harmed. When hospitals failed to take precautions and infected an ICU patient, the hospital would be paid to care for the original malady and then, on top of that, paid to fix the problem it had caused. The perversity of this incentive had long been deeply unsettling to Berwick and other leaders of the movement. IHI estimated that something on the order of 40,000 acts of harm were done to patients each day in American hospitals and, now, with the Medicare announcement, some of those—perhaps many—would not be paid for. About a month before the IHI Forum, CMS announced a pay-for-performance proposal to tie some Medicare payments to quality of care. "If you don't perform, you don't get paid as much," the acting CMS administrator, Kerry Weems, said at the time.

Perhaps the most audacious goals anywhere have been set by Ascension Health, the largest nonprofit health care organization in the country with sixty-seven hospitals and clinics spread across twenty states and the District of Columbia. Ascension has the courage to make what is perhaps the most aggressive aspirational commitment anywhere in the world of health care: A commitment to "excellent clinical care with *no preventable injuries or deaths* by July of 2008" (emphasis added). The difficulty of the challenge seems to energize the Ascension leadership. David Pryor, MD, senior vice president for clinical excellence and chief medical officer at Ascension, is working in partnership with Berwick and IHI in the nitty-gritty effort to drive the quality initiative and reach their goal. Pryor and his team are relying on the six aims enunciated in the *Chasm* report: That care will be "safe, effective, patient-centered, timely, efficient, and equitable."

Thus far, Ascension's results are impressive. After identifying the most common causes of preventable injuries and deaths, Ascension teams worked to define best practices for a variety of areas, including adverse drug events, nosocomial infections, perinatal safety, and falls. By the middle of 2005, pilot sites were reporting outcomes improved by more than 50 percent. Even more dramatically, from mid-2005 to mid-2006, "the overall mortality rate for patients not admitted for end-of-life care declined 21 percent across the system." Ascension has lower rates of pressure ulcers in its sixty-seven hospitals—93 percent below the national average, in fact; its birth injury rates are 74 percent lower, and patient falls 86 percent lower.

Ascension is one of many places drawing improvement techniques from outside health care. Just a few years ago, many clinicians scoffed at the notion that any sort of industrial quality techniques could apply in medicine, but now, throughout the country, those techniques are increasingly embraced. Gerald B. Healy, MD, otolaryngologist-in-chief at

Children's Hospital in Boston, provides a good example. Healy is a Harvard Medical School faculty member as well as president of the American College of Surgeons—an establishment figure, yet one of many who has looked outside health care for guidance. Healy discovered that commercial aviation crew management provides the consistency and dependability he wants in his OR. "Operating rooms suffer from the same flaw that once plagued cockpits," he wrote in the *Boston Globe* in early 2008. "Just as crew members had feared questioning their captains, many surgical team members still fear questioning surgeons. Many medical errors could have been avoided if a nurse, resident, or anesthesiologist had felt free to speak up. What works in the cockpit can work in the operating room." He likened pilots' standard operating procedures with evidence-based care and reported that after team training with pilots, the error rate at his hospital department dropped to zero. "As individuals, we are prone to making mistakes," he wrote, "but as part of high-performance teams, we can avoid or minimize those mistakes."

An important thread woven through the tapestry of change that Paul Batalden refers to involves significant reform of education and training for medical students and residents. If medical students are introduced to the world of quality improvement—if they learn how to apply improvement skills early on—they will be much more effective during their years of practice. Just as Batalden believed that the Joint Commission was a crucial pressure point in spreading the improvement gospel throughout American hospitals, he believes that another credentialing body, the Accreditation Council for Graduate Medical Education (ACGME), which accredits 8,200 residency programs educating 100,000-plus residents, can play a pivotal role by requiring improvement instruction for students. For a number of years, Batalden worked with David Leach, MD, the former executive director of ACGME and Leach met with considerable success in changing the curriculum to require improvement capabilities.

"When I was training it was really an apprentice program," says Leach. "I tagged along and was expected to imitate faculty and from that develop my own style of practice." Under new ACGME accreditation rules, however, students must demonstrate competencies in the areas of patient care, medical knowledge, professionalism, interpersonal and communications skills, practice-based learning and improvement, and system-based practice.

"By and large doctors are system illiterate," observes Leach. "They don't see the system." But if they learn in training how to see care as a system issue—see practice as a team effort—it will make them much more amenable to system-based quality improvement. Think of the impact, says Batalden, when 100,000 residents per year go through training that enables them to work within systems as team players applying quality improvement skills. In just a decade, that equals 1 million doctors trained in quality improvement.

The new quality movement is improving care for millions of patients throughout the world, an historic achievement to be celebrated for years to come.

But it is also an achievement that advances the movement toward its next phase—an immensely challenging frontier. Berwick defines the challenge as the Triple Aim: First, provide high quality care for individuals—the area where the movement has achieved such important strides; second, improve the health of populations; and third, reduce the per capita cost of care.

Such a prosaic term as Triple Aim hardly does justice to what is more aptly described as the Holy Grail of health care. Fixing quality and safety and then maintaining the health of populations while reducing the per capita cost of care—this is a grand and worthy vision. It is also an urgent challenge in the face of ever-rising health care costs that threaten to strangle the U.S. economy. So how can the Grail be found?

We need to devise and then implement on a broad scale payment methods that reward providers for quality and appropriateness rather than volume and complexity. We need to shift from the current model where we typically pay for volume, complexity, and intensity to paying for outcomes (quality) and appropriateness (efficiency). Fundamentally, we need to change the financing system so that providers are paid for the care of populations rather than for hospitalization or procedures. This was the original HMO model in its purest form, says Berwick, "before it got tarred and feathered by mutant forms that took the name but not the heart of it." The difficulty is how best to manage population-based care when the financial structure not only does not provide incentives for quality, but quite often sets up unintentionally perverse quality *disincentives*. Aligning incentives with quality outcomes is essential. If promoting the health of a population is in the financial interest of a hospital or physician practice the result is healthier patients who avoid hospitalization. Reducing hospital use is essential to controlling costs, yet Berwick observes that "our whole system is structured the other way. We celebrate high occupancy rates and growth of use." Only half jokingly, Berwick suggests that the best way to recognize that the Holy Grail is within reach would be hospitals "trying to be emptier, not fuller."

The system as it stands is badly out of balance: The vast majority of resources, time, and talent go into caring for people when they get sick as opposed to bringing to bear resources, time, and talent to prevent them from getting sick or, when they do (in the case of chronic illnesses) helping them manage their conditions so they do not deteriorate to the point where they require hospitalization.

The conflict that must be resolved to find the Holy Grail is embedded deeply within the DNA of the American health care system. Hospitals strive for full beds, but hospital admissions are gasoline on the fire of rising costs. And many hospitalized patients—those with chronic illnesses, typically—are there because the system has already failed them; failed to provide preventive care, for example, or failed to provide the kind of routine maintenance care that keeps patients' chronic conditions under control.

The notion of paying for quality rather than a series of functions is gaining traction in part as a result of work by Michael E. Porter, the renowned Harvard Business School professor. Porter argues that improving the quality of care can reduce costs, and he observes that every other major sector of the economy with the exception of health care has undergone reconfiguration. Health care, says Porter, would benefit from measurement and competition and a structure where physicians are rewarded for value—and value in health care means *quality at a reasonable cost.*

This new phase of the quality movement presents immensely complex challenges. Reaching the grail will require consummate skill, powers of persuasion and an unrelenting nature. As difficult as it will be, there is no question it is achievable. Who would bet against Berwick and the force that has already accomplished so much and created a powerful momentum for change? Who would bet against the 6,000-plus delegates at the Forum? Who would bet against this movement?

When Berwick appeared on stage in Orlando for his annual speech to the Forum delegates, he looked out over a vast convention center where thousands awaited his words. These events have taken on a somewhat mythic feel through the years as time after time Berwick has spun long, engaging yarns about the movement, tying seemingly disparate elements together in beautiful rhetorical packages. His speeches, in fact, have generally been so good that eleven of them were published in book form in 2004 under the title *Escape Fire.* Typically, they weave elements of story-telling, inspiration and vision in almost equal measure. This year, though, he tells the assembled multitudes that he has something different. Berwick says that he shared a draft of his speech with a colleague who had an interesting response. The colleague told Berwick that he had gone to a Bruce Springsteen concert a while back and at the beginning of the show Springsteen had come on stage and told the audience that he planned to play new songs and not the old favorites he knew fans wanted to hear. But the singer asked the audience to give him a chance with the new material, and they did. Berwick read between the lines and said the message he took from his friend's comment was: "Don, this speech is a problem. People expect "Thunder Road," and this ain't it. Better warn them." He said he had something more "wonky and technical" than usual. And, to some extent, it was just that. Berwick burrowed deeply into a discussion of the nature of medical research and the relative merits of studies of varying depth and complexity.

But he did not abandon "Thunder Road" altogether for contained within his speech—wrapped under a few layers of policy discussion—was an unmistakable battle cry. He urged action. He urged them to do more, to *go faster*. Millions of patients were depending upon the men and women of the movement to work intelligently and quickly to find new and better ways to deliver treatments. Historically in medicine, change too often was propelled only by detailed scientific studies. He cautioned delegates against becoming paralyzed by *Primum non nocere* (first, do no harm), which Berwick said is generally interpreted as "don't change the status quo unless you're sure." He challenged delegates to "reconsider our attitudes toward thresholds for action. When do we wait for more knowledge? And when do we go ahead, pull the trigger, *act*?"

Berwick has been at this for thirty-plus years now, and all the achievements have still not made him entirely comfortable about sitting squarely within the establishment. He still relishes his role as a kind of outsider. "The status quo isn't very attractive; it's ugly," he declares. "So, do we actually *want* to give the status quo such a leg up?"

Instead of *primum non nocere,* he suggests, what about, maybe, *"primum, don't just stand there?"*

He envisioned a global network of experimentation yielding new best practices at every level of care; a network where tens of thousands of clinicians engaged in a sustained effort to learn from one another for the benefit of millions of patients around the world. Berwick pressed the audience:

> [P]roceed urgently to test promising changes, and, as you do that, gather evidence to guide further choices and broader implementation. That way, we can learn much faster than if we wait for truth to emerge only from formal research processes conducted by only a few among us.
>
> Improvement, properly done, *is* research and learning. And, widespread improvement is widespread research. Think of it. Local knowledge is now growing every day in thousands of settings as hundreds of thousands of clinicians, managers, and others, learn. . . . This way to learn isn't the same as delegating research to a small segment of the health care industry. We ought to be, not a small network of professional laboratories, but an immense network for a learning community. Formal science, housed in formal research centers, should remain preeminent in supplying new ideas and technologies—hard, cold facts; but local improvement can be common, continual, disciplined, and informative to all.
>
> This is urgent: to expand our vision with more inclusive, but no less disciplined commitments to science and evidence. It is urgent because our aim is so much grander than a good trial well-published. Our aim is progress against the suffering.

And no sooner was the conference concluded in Orlando than Berwick was off—on airplanes traveling in various directions, crisscrossing the country, promoting the 5 *Million Lives* campaign while simultaneously pursuing the Holy Grail.

Though unintentional, there is a certain irony to the conclusion of the 5 *Million Lives* campaign because it falls in December of 2008, fourteen years—nearly to the day—after the death of Betsy Lehman. If the Institute of Medicine is correct, anywhere from 700,000 to nearly 1.5 million people have died from preventable medical errors since Betsy lost her life. These are staggering numbers in the aggregate, but each one is a separate story, a separate world in a way. Consider the magnitude of the loss of Betsy Lehman to her husband and daughters, to her mother, friends, and colleagues. Or the unspeakable loss of Josie King to Sorrel and Tony. Or the death of Josh for Victoria and Armando Nahum. Each of these individual cases is an epic unto itself, and these are but three examples from a universe of harm. They represent perhaps as little as one thousandth of 1 percent.

And if the IHI is correct in its numbers—that there are approximately 15 million instances of medical harm in the United States each year, that amounts to 210 million harmful events since Betsy died. Even in a time when we are often numb to statistics, that number—or even a half of it or a quarter of it—is a heartbreaking toll.

But then, that is the beauty of this movement, of this event in Orlando where, upon its completion, Berwick and the other 6,000-plus go off to thousands of destinations around the world determined to change those numbers; determined to prevent that harm. And given what they have accomplished already, who is to say they will not triumph?

Notes

INTRODUCTION

The introduction relies upon the extensive coverage of Betsy Lehman's death by former colleagues at the *Boston Globe*. I relied in particular on work by former *Globe* staff writers Dick Lehr and Richard A. Knox. A Knox article of March 23, 1995—"Doctor's Orders Killed Cancer Patient"—was particularly informative. And an article by Lehr the same day—"I Think the Human Touch Means Everything"—provided excerpts from Betsy's correspondence with friends. I also relied upon Harvard Business School case studies on the Dana-Farber Cancer nstitute by R. Bohmer and A. Winslow, Dana-Farber Cancer Institute, Harvard Business School Publishing, 1999; also R. Bohmer, Dana-Farber Cancer Institute; Harvard Business School Teaching Note 603–092; Harvard Business School Publishing, 2003. Information for the introduction came from the two landmark Institute of Medicine studies—*To Err Is Human: Building a Safer Health System* (National Academy Press, 2000) by editors Linda T. Kohn, Janet M. Corrigan, and Molla S. Donaldson; and *Crossing the Quality Chasm: A New*

Health System for the 21st Century (National Academy Press, 2001) by Janet M. Corrigan, project director. I also relied upon a *Time* magazine article, "The Disturbing Case of the Cure That Killed the Patient," by Christine Gorman, April 3, 1994. Other articles I relied upon include "We Can Do Better—Improving the Health of the American People" by Steven A. Schroeder, MD, published in the *New England Journal of Medicine* 357, no. 12 (September 20, 2007): 1221–1228. For various data I relied upon both RAND work by Beth McGlynn et al., the Commonwealth Fund, and the National Committee for Quality Assurance. For insight and guidance on the introduction, I relied upon interviews with Don Berwick, Maureen Bisognano, Jim Conway, and George Halvorson. I relied also on "Redefining Health Care" by Michael E. Porter and Elizabeth Olmstead Teisberg.

CHAPTER 1

Chapter 1 relies heavily on extensive interviews with Don Berwick as well as interviews with Paul Batalden. Berwick's book *Escape Fire* provided much information, particularly concerning the anecdotes focused on Guy Cohen and NASA. For information on W. Edwards Deming, I relied upon discussions with Berwick and Batalden as well as upon Mary Walton's book *Deming Management At Work* (1991) and Deming's book *Out of the Crisis* (1982).

CHAPTER 2

Chapter 2 relies on interviews with Don Berwick; Maureen Bisognano; Paul Batalden; Blan Godfrey, PhD; Gene Nelson, PhD; Tom Nolan, PhD, James Roberts, MD, Dave Gustafson, PhD, Vinod K. Sahney, PhD; and James Schlosser, MD, MBA. The chapter relies as well on interviews with Dick Sharpe, formerly of the John A. Hartford Foundation, which funded the National Demonstration Project. The chapter relies as well on the book *Curing Health Care: New*

Strategies for Quality Improvement by Berwick, Blan Godfrey, and Jane Roessner (Jossey-Bass 1990).

CHAPTER 3

The chapter relies heavily on a series of interviews with Lucian Leape, MD. It also relies on an interview with Howard Hiatt, MD, former dean of the Harvard School of Public Health. It relies as well on an article by Leape and Troy Brennan, MD, "Error in Medicine," published in *JAMA* (December 1994), as well as the article "Incidence of Adverse Drug Events and Potential Adverse Drug Events, and Systems Analysis of Adverse Drug Events" by Leape and David Bates, MD, *Journal of the American Medical Association* 274 (1995): 29–43. The chapter also relies on the text of the speech Leape gave to the Annenberg conference on error. The chapter relies upon a series of articles in the *New England Journal of Medicine* by David Blumenthal, MD, and others on quality care.

CHAPTER 4

The chapter relies upon interviews with Berwick and Janet Corrigan. It also relies on discussions with Beth McGlynn from RAND as well as the text of McGlynn's testimony to the presidential commission (based on work conducted at RAND by McGlynn, Bob Brook, Mark Schuster, et al.). The chapter relies upon a June 2003 article in the *New England Journal of Medicine* titled "The Quality of Health Care Delivered to Adults in the United States" by McGlynn writing with RAND colleagues Steven M. Asch, MD; John Adams, PhD; Joan Keesey; Jennifer Hicks, MPH, PhD; Alison DeCristofaro, MPH; and Eve A. Kerr, MD, MPH. The chapter also draws from the two major IOM reports: *To Err* and *Chasm*. The chapter draws from various news articles, including those published in the *Washington Post* by Rick Weiss, November 30, 1999; in the *Wall Street Journal* by Ron Winslow, November 30, 1999;

and in the *New York Times* by Sheryl Gay Stolberg, December 5, 1999. It relies as well on an article by Mark R. Chassin, MD, in the *Millbank Quarterly* 76, no. 4 (1998): 565–591. The chapter relies on a study by researchers from the Harvard School of Public Health and the Kaiser Family Foundation into attitudes of physicians and the public toward the findings in "To Err Is Human," *New England Journal of Medicine* 347, no. 24 (December 2, 2002): 1993–1940.

CHAPTER 5

This chapter relies largely on interviews with Rick Shannon. It also draws from an interview with Paul O'Neill and from information contained on the Web site of the Pittsburgh Regional Health Initiative. It relies as well on articles in the *Pittsburgh Post-Gazette* by Christopher Snowbeck, December 2, 2002, and Gary Rotstein, December 30, 2003.

CHAPTER 6

The chapter relies upon information derived from interviews with Uma Kotagal, Jim Anderson, and Lee Carter. The chapter also relies upon interviews with Don Berwick as well as a number of Cincinnati Children's physicians, including Maria Britto, Fred Ryckman, Keith Mandel, and Steve Muething. The chapter draws from interviews with Tom Nolan, PhD, and Maureen Bisognano of IHI. The chapter relies upon the *New Yorker* article "The Bell Curve: What Happens When Patients Find Out How Good Their Doctors Really Are?" by Atul Gawande, MD, published December 6, 2004.

CHAPTER 7

The chapter relies on interviews with Gary Kaplan, MD, and Mike Rona, former president of Virginia Mason, as well as on interviews with Drs. Robert Caplan, Robert Mecklenburg, and Fred Govier. The chapter also relies upon interviews with Charleen Tachibana, Chief Nursing Officer; Sarah Patterson, Executive Vice President; Cathie Furman, RN, MHA, Vice President of Quality and Compliance; Kathleen Paul, Chief of Communications; Deb Heinricher, RN; and Denise Dubuque, Administrative Director of the Cancer Institute. The chapter also relies on interviews with Don Berwick and Art Byrne, former CEO of Wiremold. The chapter relies on the book *A World Class Production System* by John R. Black; and on the *Seattle Times,* including an article by Lisa Heyamoto, June 6, 2002. It relies as well on a Harvard Business School study of Virginia Mason. Information for the chapter is drawn from the *New York Times* of January 11, 2006. It relies as well on *Today's Hospitalist* magazine.

CHAPTER 8

The chapter is based in large part on interviews with Sorrel King. It relies as well on an excellent two-part series of articles in the *Baltimore Sun* by Erika Niedowski called "A Mother's Promise: How Medical Errors Took a Little Girl's Life," published on December 14, 2003. It relies on information from the University of Pittsburgh Medical Center Web site, and on Lucian Leape's presentation "When Things Go Wrong," from May 2006. It relies also on an interview with Armando and Victoria Nahum.

CHAPTER 9

The chapter relies on interviews with Göran Henriks, Mats Bojestig, MD, and Sven Olof Karlsson. It also relies upon interviews with Don Berwick, Maureen Bisognano, Paul Batalden, and Brent James, MD. Information is derived from *Diffusion of Innovations* by E. M. Rogers, and from Berwick's *Escape Fire*. Information was also derived from articles in the publication *Quality Management in Health Care* 16, no. 1 (January/March 2007): "Making Systemwide

Improvements in Health Care: Lessons From Jönköping County, Sweden" by Thomas Bodenheimer, MD; Mats Bojestig, MD, PhD; and Göran Henriks, MBA. And "The Health Care Quality Journey of Jönköping County Council, Sweden" by Boel Andersson-Gäre, MD, PhD; and Duncan Neuhauser, PhD.

CHAPTER 10

The chapter relies on interviews with George Halvorson as well as others at Kaiser, including Drs. Louise Liang, Andy Wiesenthal and Mark Groshek. It relies on Alida Chase, Anna-Lisa Silvestre, Holly Potter, Jack Cochran, Ruth Brentani, and John August. It relies as well on discussions with Don Berwick and Maureen Bisognano. The chapter relies on George Halvorson's books *Health Care Reform Now! A Prescription for Change* (2007); and *Epidemic of Care: A Call for Safer, Better and More Accountable Health Care* (2003) (coauthored by George J. Isham, MD). The chapter draws from the *New York Times*, particularly "Smart Care Via a Mouse, But What Will It Cost?" by Steve Lohr, published August 20, 2006. The chapter relies also on a discussion with Ronald Paulus of Geisinger Health System.

CHAPTER 11

The chapter relies on interviews with Don Berwick; Paul Batalden; Maureen Bisognano; and David Leach, MD. I rely upon interviews with Commonwealth Fund leaders Karen Davis, PhD, and Steve Schoenbaum, MD. I also rely upon two reports produced by the Commonwealth Fund Commission on a High Performance Health System: Framework for a High Performance Health System in the United States (August 2006), and Bending the Curve: Options for Achieving Savings and Improving Value in U.S. Health Spending (December 2007). I rely upon "Redefining Health Care" by Porter and Teisberg. Material was drawn from a *US News* interview with

Berwick as well as from *Modern Healthcare, Health Affairs,* and the *Boston Globe*. Information was drawn from *Ascension Health*. Information about awards to Berwick was drawn from the Association of University Programs in Health Administration (AUPHA) and from the Baxter International Foundation, which awards the William B. Graham Prize for Health Services Research. I rely upon *Measuring the Health of Nations: Updating an Earlier Analysis,* published in *Health Affairs* (January–February 2008). Additional information was drawn from The Doctors Company.

ADDITIONAL NOTE ON SOURCES

I rely upon the thinking and writings of a number of other individuals and organizations, including: Dennis O'Leary, MD, former president of the Joint Commission; Troy Brennan, MD; David Bates, MD; Joseph Juran; James Reason, author of *Human Error*; David Blumenthal, MD, and Jack Wennberg, MD; Elliott Fisher, MD, and colleagues at Dartmouth for their landmark work on variation. I was informed by the PBS series "Remaking American Medicine," and by the work of William C. Richardson, leader of the two major IOM committees; Mark R. Chassin, MD, president of the Joint Commission, and Robert W. Galvin for their work on the IOM National Roundtable on Health Care Quality; David Lawrence, MD, former CEO of Kaiser Permanente ("The chassis is broken"); Molly Joel Coye, MD; Lonnie R. Bristow, MD, former president of the AMA; George J. Isham, MD; Professor Brian Jarman, PhD; Linda Kenney; Sister Mary Jean Ryan; Steve Jencks, MD; the Robert Wood Johnson Foundation; the National Quality Forum; the National Committee for Quality Assurance; the National Patient Safety Foundation, and the Commonwealth Fund.

It is important to recognize the contributions of pioneers whose work the new quality movement built upon. (For this historical summary I rely upon Brennan and Berwick's "New Rules: Regulation, Markets, and the Quality of American Health Care.) Although Deming played a fundamental role in influencing Berwick and Batalden during the 1980s and beyond, there were other thinkers whose work laid the foundation for the new quality movement, including Ernest Codman, a surgeon at Massachusetts General Hospital, Boston, between 1900 and 1920, who was the first to see the study of quality in medicine as an area for scientific inquiry. In the 1940s and 1950s, Paul Lembcke, a surgeon at Johns Hopkins Hospital, went beyond Codman in attempting to establish ways to collect and analyze data to detect and learn from clinical practice variation. In 1966, one of the most important papers on health care quality ever written was published by Avedis Donabedian, MD, of the University of Michigan, called "Evaluating the Quality of Medical Care." During the 1960s, landmark quality work was conducted at Johns Hopkins and the Yale University School of Medicine, among others. At Hopkins, Kerr White, MD, chairman of medicine, and John Williamson, MD, began to see that industrial quality techniques might apply to health care. Williamson mentored Bob Brook, a Hopkins medical student, who would go on to lead the RAND work on health care quality, contributing a substantive, data-driven foundation that all future quality advocates would build upon. During the 1970s, Jack Wennberg, MD, conducted breakthrough research relating to quality. Along with his colleague Alan Gittelsohn, Wennberg published a paper on variations in clinical practice patterns throughout the country in 1973 in the journal *Science*. Wennberg and Gittelsohn found large variations in health care usage in various parts of the country; they noted that in communities employing a large number of thoracic surgeons the incidence of thoracic surgery was higher than in other communities. The disturbing pattern they found was that treatments seemed driven by supply rather than demand. These variations were not explained by, as Wennberg put it, "illness, patient preference, or the dictates of evidence-based medicine." (See *Physicians for a National Health Program Web site:* "Practice Variations and Health Care Reform: Connecting the Dots," by John E. Wennberg, October 7, 2004.)

Acknowledgments

This book is a product in large measure of the generosity—with their time, insights and ideas—of scores of men and women throughout the health care universe. I was welcomed into this world by clinicians, scholars, administrators, and others eager to share their thinking and more than willing to explain their work. These tend to be exceptionally busy people, yet whenever I asked for time to discuss various issues the answer was always in the affirmative. Having access to the brain-power that populates the quality movement made this book possible.

I am grateful to the early pioneers from the Birthday Club including Gene Nelson, PhD; Dave Gustafson, PhD; Vinod K. Sahney, PhD; James Schlosser, MD, MBA; and James Roberts, MD, who read drafts of the Birthday Club section and provided important guidance. Vin Sahney also reviewed early chapters. Thanks go to Blanton Godfrey, PhD, former head of Bell Labs Quality Theory and Technology Department; Howard Hiatt, MD, former dean of the Harvard School of Public Health; Janet Corrigan, PhD, staff director on both *To Err* and *Chasm*; to Paul O'Neill, the former secretary of the treasury; Diane Pinakiewicz at the National Patient Safety Foundation; Ben Sachs, MD, formerly of BI Deaconess in Boston; Ron

Paulus, MD, at Geisinger; and Rashad Massoud, MD, formerly at IHI. I enjoyed thoughtful discussions about physician compacts with the experts: Jack Silversin, DDS, and Mary Jane Kornacki. Thanks to Karen Davis, PhD, and Steve Schoenbaum, MD, of the Commonwealth Fund; and to David Leach, MD, former executive director of ACGME. I owe a debt of gratitude to David Pryor, MD, chief medical officer at Ascension, for spending a morning with me in St. Louis during which he enunciated the most daring goals anywhere in health care. Thanks to Jim Reinertsen, MD, one of the more brilliant communicators within the movement. A special thanks to Brent James, MD, from Intermountain for sharing his thoughts and for his remarkable work through the decades.

The substantive basis for this book would likely not exist were it not for the landmark work of the people at RAND, particularly Bob Brook, MD, and Beth McGlynn, PhD; and their colleagues.

Rick Shannon, MD, brings a striking passion and intensity to his work and I thank him for his time and guidance.

I am deeply grateful to the team at Cincinnati Children's. My visits there were as pleasurable as they were instructive thanks to Drs. Maria Britto, Keith Mandel, Steve Muething, Fred Ryckman, and Kim Pittenger. I appreciate the help from Kathy Dressman, Scott Hamlin, Linda Morris, and Steve Campbell. Thanks go to Jim Anderson, the Cincinnati CEO, and Lee Carter, chairman of the board— good people doing great work. Finally at Cincinnati, it is an honor to play a role in telling the story of Dr. Uma Kotagal, a true guiding light within the quality movement.

Many people at Virginia Mason Medical Center in Seattle provided important help and guidance, including Charleen Tachibana, chief nursing officer; Sarah Patterson, executive vice president; Cathie Furman, RN, MHA, vice president of quality and compliance; Deb Heinricher, RN; Denise Dubuque; Christina Saint Martin; Neil B. Hampson, MD; Linda Hebish; and Dick Foley. I would also like to thank Fred Govier,

MD, chief of surgery; the ever-professional Kathleen Paul, chief of communications; and Mike Rona, former president. I received important insights about the Toyota Production System from Art Byrne, former CEO of Wiremold, as well as from Dr. Robert Caplan. I am very grateful to Robert Mecklenburg, MD, former chief of medicine at Virginia Mason. My greatest debt at Virginia Mason, of course, is to Gary Kaplan, MD, the CEO. He has embarked on an exciting and courageous journey.

I am profoundly grateful to Sorrel and Tony King for sharing their incredibly painful story. I am grateful as well to Armando and Victoria Nahum for sharing theirs.

Unusually gracious hosts are to be found in Jönköping County, Sweden, where my colleague Robert Mandel, MD, and I received the warmest of welcomes. Sven Olof Karlsson, CEO of the County Council; Göran Henriks, chief of learning and innovation; and Mats Bojestig, MD, PhD, chief medical officer, were generous with their time and insights. We also wish to thank the amiable staff at Qulturum, especially Kerstin Arnell. We are grateful to Dr. Raymond Lenrick, chief of obstetrics and gynecology; Boel Andersson-Gäre, MD, PhD; and, of course, to Esther.

At Kaiser Permanente I am most grateful for their time and insights to Louise Liang, MD; Alida Chase; Anna-Lisa Silvestre; Jack Corcoran, MD; Ruth Brentani; John August; Andy Wiesenthal, MD; and Mark Groshek, MD. Holly Potter is an expert in communications and I owe her a debt for her professionalism and for going above and beyond the call. Finally at Kaiser, I am indebted to the affable, thoughtful—and very wise—George Halvorson.

It is important to acknowledge the work done by former colleagues of mine at the *Boston Globe* in writing about the death of Betsy Lehman. Many staffers at the *Globe* did good work, but I particularly want to acknowledge the contribution of two former colleagues—both having moved on from the *Globe*—Dick Lehr and Richard A. Knox. I want to thank as well Don Aucoin and Lisa Tuite of the *Globe* for reviewing a portion of the manuscript and providing important editorial suggestions.

I am indebted to Lucian Leape, MD, for his help, particularly concerning medical errors, a field in which he is the acknowledged worldwide expert.

At the Institute for Healthcare Improvement in Cambridge I owe many more debts than I can ever repay. Thanks go to Dan Schummers; Markus Josephson; Tom Nolan, PhD, Andrea Kabcanell, Jonathan Small, Madge Kaplan, and Jane Roessner. Jim Conway helped launch me on this journey, and Maureen Bisognano helped me stay the course with her encouragement and by smart suggestions in so many areas. The same goes for Paul Batalden. Like Uma, Maureen and Paul are among the real guiding lights of the movement. Finally at IHI, Don Berwick was generous, kind, patient, and always insightful. This story would not exist without Don.

I am blessed by my association with the consummate professionals at PublicAffairs. I feel most fortunate, once again, to feel the embrace of Susan Weinberg, Peter Osnos, Robert Kimzey, Lisa Kaufman, Whitney Peeling, and Clive Priddle—a great team of serious publishers. I am grateful to Dan Ozzi and Lindsay Goodman. And I owe more than I can say to my editor, Niki Papadopoulos, whose deft, intelligent fingerprints are all over these pages. She made this a much better book.

Throughout the process I received support from my family—my wife Anne, son Charlie and daughter Elizabeth. I am grateful to my friend Charles A. Tracy, MD, for his informal tutorials through the years about the practice of medicine. He inspired me throughout this process.

Finally, I owe an enormous debt to my friends and colleagues at Blue Cross Blue Shield of Massachusetts, where I am privileged to serve as a consultant on the quality initiative. When I first mentioned the idea of writing this book to Peter Meade and John Schoenbaum, they were immediately supportive and enthusiastic and they granted me the leeway to work on the book while working on other Blue

Cross projects. John served as godfather to the book in many ways and it would not have happened without him. Also at Blue Cross I received intelligent and deft guidance from Andrew Dreyfus; Fredi Shonkoff; Vin Sahney, PhD (a Birthday Club member now at Blue Cross); Hilary McCarthy, and Audrey Shelto. Robert Mandel, MD, MBA, played a pivotal advisory role throughout. I also received support from John Fallon, MD, and from Ralph Martin, a friend and a member of the Blue Cross Board of Directors. I am grateful to Nancy Driscoll for her professionalism and hard work, and I thank Eric Menn as well. Finally, I owe an enduring debt of gratitude to Cleve L. Killingsworth, CEO at Blue Cross. Cleve brings a combination of passion and intellectual rigor to the quality movement and has emerged as one of the most important figures in the movement in the United States. I am grateful for his leadership and support.

Index

‒‒‒‒‒‒‒‒

Furman, Cathie, 184–185
Future of the quality movement,
276–279

G

Galvin, Robert W., 80
Gawande, Atul, 18, 147–150
Geisinger Health System, 258, 259,
277
Genie Industries, 168, 170
Gingrich, Newt, 269
Godfrey, Blanton, 40–41, 45, 223
Gonsalves, Gerry, 24
Govier, Fred, 170–171, 185–186
Greenberg, Ann. *See* Berwick, Ann
Groshek, Mark, 255–256, 260
Gustafson, Dave, 48, 50, 223

H

Halvorson, George, 11, 274
books by, 239–240
Cerner and Epic systems and,
250–254
on chronic diseases, 241
educational background of,
237–238
evidence-based care and, 242
on financial incentives, 261–263
interest in health care quality
improvement, 239–241, 263
joins Kaiser Permanente,
242–244
personal health issues, 252

technology changes made by,
247–250
Hartford Foundation, 40
Harvard Community Health Plan,
15–17, 20–21, 35, 41, 48
compared to NASA, 22–25
Hatlie, Martin, 67
Health Care Co-Ops in Uganda
(Halvorson), 240
Health care Reform (Halvorson),
239
Healthcare Corporation of
America, 33, 45, 48, 50
Healthcare Today (journal), 261
Healy, Gerald B., 278–279
Heinricher, Deb, 187
Henriks, Göran, 216, 239
Balanced Scorecard approach,
220–222
educational background of, 218
health care quality improvement
and, 222–228
patient centered care and,
229–230
Herman, Alexis, 74
Hippocrates, 7
Hospital Quality Alliance, 275
Hospitals
clinical effectiveness programs,
129–130
current quality improvement
efforts by, 276–279
Electronic Medical Records, 92,
214
emergency room services, 42, 153
financial incentives and,
261–263, 280–282

Q

Quality, health care
Balanced Scorecard approach,
220–222
billing errors and, 41–42, 92–93
changing, 13
Commonwealth Fund and,
273–275
continuous improvement,
46–47
costs of care and, 280–282
defined, 7–8, 65–66, 100
Deming approach and, 27–37
evidence-based care and, 91–92,
151–152, 242, 279
financial incentives and,
261–263
future of, 276–279
information technology and,
89–93, 241, 244–263
Institute for Healthcare
Improvement and, 10, 17–18,
55–60, 265–273
media coverage of, 84, 86–88,
102–103, 108–111, 147–148,
171–172
National Demonstration Project,
40–51
patient-centered care and,
228–235
patient safety alerts and,
180–185
patients' views on, 44–45
performance measurements and,
10–12, 241–242

President's Advisory Commission
on Consumer Protection and
Quality and, 74–75
preventive care and, 9, 233–234,
282
public interest in, 84–88
spending and, 8–9
studies on, 7–12, 75–80
threshold improvement in, 79
top-down change and, 226–228
Toyota Production System
applied to, 100–101,
104–105
transparency and, 108–111,
155–156, 210–211
See also Physicians
*Quality Assurance in Ambulatory
Care* (Batalden), 27
Quality First (President's Advisory
Commission on Consumer
Protection and Quality in the
Health Care Industry), 78
*Quality Management in Health
Care* (journal), 235
Qulturum, 217–218, 234–235

R

RAND Corporation, 7, 9–10, 48,
62–63, 75, 94–95, 273
Rapid response teams, hospital,
206–207
Reinertsen, James L., 89
"Remaking American Medicine,"
147

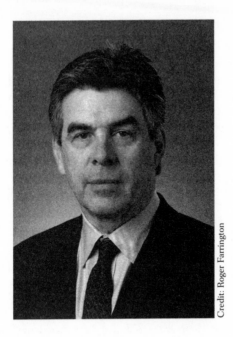

Credit: Roger Farrington

Charles Kenney is an author, consultant and former journalist at the *Boston Globe*. Among his nonfiction books are *John F. Kennedy: The Presidential Portfolio,* and *Rescue Men.* He is also the author of the novels *Hammurabi's Code, The Son of John Devlin,* and *The Last Man.* In addition to his work as an author he serves as a consultant to Blue Cross Blue Shield of Massachusetts on the company's quality and safety initiative. He lives in Boston, Massachusetts.

PublicAffairs is a publishing house founded in 1997. It is a tribute to the standards, values, and flair of three persons who have served as mentors to countless reporters, writers, editors, and book people of all kinds, including me.

I. F. Stone, proprietor of *I. F. Stone's Weekly*, combined a commitment to the First Amendment with entrepreneurial zeal and reporting skill and became one of the great independent journalists in American history. At the age of eighty, Izzy published *The Trial of Socrates*, which was a national bestseller. He wrote the book after he taught himself ancient Greek.

Benjamin C. Bradlee was for nearly thirty years the charismatic editorial leader of *The Washington Post*. It was Ben who gave the *Post* the range and courage to pursue such historic issues as Watergate. He supported his reporters with a tenacity that made them fearless and it is no accident that so many became authors of influential, best-selling books.

Robert L. Bernstein, the chief executive of Random House for more than a quarter century, guided one of the nation's premier publishing houses. Bob was personally responsible for many books of political dissent and argument that challenged tyranny around the globe. He is also the founder and longtime chair of Human Rights Watch, one of the most respected human rights organizations in the world.

·　　·　　·

For fifty years, the banner of Public Affairs Press was carried by its owner Morris B. Schnapper, who published Gandhi, Nasser, Toynbee, Truman, and about 1,500 other authors. In 1983, Schnapper was described by *The Washington Post* as "a redoubtable gadfly." His legacy will endure in the books to come.